HIGH ANXIETY

A search for evidence-based interventions

Exclusive Copyright: Klaus Kuch, MD
February 8, 2022

To Wendy,
my vastly better half

1. How it all started
2. Which end is up?
3. Pot, booze and snowbirds
4. Learning to feel: Esalen and the Student Health Service
5. A very different scene: Toronto, Ontario
6. On staff at last
7. First dips: Investigating a headache
8. High anxiety, in the skies and elsewhere
9. Social phobia: What will people think?
10. The many faces of posttraumatic stress disorder
11. The horror of the Nazi concentration camps
12. The misery of chronic pain
13. Why the fuss about science?
14. There really is a Kalamazoo
15. Other research
16. Sweating it in Court
17. The rubber chicken circuit
18. Who's next?
19. The rant
20. Before I go

21. Abbreviations
22. References and recommendations for further reading

INTRODUCTION

I never planned it his way. Illness preempted a pathology career in my native Germany. Curiosity inspired a move to the Southern USA, later to Canada. I took a University job there in Toronto and stayed. After a foray into Gestalt therapy, phobias, panic anxiety and PTSD became focal points in my psychiatric practice, later also chronic pain. Doubts about the effectiveness of psychotherapy had me investigate physiological markers of distress. That didn't succeed, but behavior therapy did with anxious survivors of car accidents, with animal phobias, social fears, fear of flying and agoraphobia. Drug research deepened my knowledge of objective assessment methods and opened up more questions. What slows the recovery from accidents and assaults? How do agoraphobics fare after completing drug and behavior therapy? What is disablement and what turns pain into chronic pain and pain disability?

Court cases require objectivity similar to research, notably in cases that pit psychiatric experts with different theoretical orientations against each other about the nature of psychological trauma and its influence on allegedly criminal acts. Several of the court cases described here were precedent-setting. Many were also emotionally challenging, especially the assessments of Nazi concentration camp survivors conducted on behalf of German courts and some Canadian cases conducted in the glare of publicity.

How does a babe from the woods acquire the necessary know-how? That's the main part of the story, the one that matters to everyone. What does an objective assessment look like? How can we measure anxiety and pain, and how can that improve self-help and clinical care? What are reinforcers and feedback loops, and what role do they play in human behavior? What's the "null-hypothesis," and how can it inform debate? The same skills that enable research can help us confront speculation and misinformation. Research provided the methods, and court battles tested them many times over.

Most of my refereed publications can be found on semanticscholar.com and researchgate.net.

Naturally I have a few opinions about all this after four decades of practice. But opinions have short legs. Just look at the history of medicine and see how few cherished "truths" have survived the last fifty years. Only the how-to of objective observation, description and evaluation has stood the test of time. That's my key point. Scientific know-how is our antidote against fake cures and fake news. "How did you arrive at your opinion" is the key question we need to pose. We need to pose it routinely and repeatedly, in regards to health care and just about everywhere else.

I have revised the original manuscript of "Medical Migrant" (published in December 2019) with the vaccine debate in mind, to describe more clearly the larger themes within my story. You can read it fast and you can read it slow, pick a chapter according to interest or read it in sequence, read it to be amused or informed. Clinical psychiatry can be as practical as plumbing, many of its techniques useful to just about everyone. I'd be gratified if my story demonstrates this even to a small extent.

Any writing about health care needs a disclaimer. I'll give you three.

- This is a story about one doctor's experiences with medical school, clinical psychiatry, research and the Courts. I want it to be useful, but it isn't advice. If you need advice, please ask your doctor or lawyer.

- Its descriptions of an autopsy, of abuse and assault may not be for the faint of heart or those who fear being "triggered."
- I write this from memory after fifteen years of retirement. And even I make the occasional mistake (according to my spouse).

1.HOW IT STARTED

According to an old folk tale all babies await their delivery in a pond called the Kinderteich (the babies' pond). They splash about until the stork arrives, bundles them up and delivers them to a random destination where overjoyed parents await. Actual procreation may look different, but the Kinderteich is spot-on in another way. It illustrates the lottery of birth and the irrationality of pride based solely on race and nationality. Being born into and nurtured by a great nation is plain old luck, not an accomplishment worth waving flags about. I had no choice in the matter when the stork deposited my bundle smack into the middle of WWII to two small-town doctors in Southern Germany. I could have done worse.

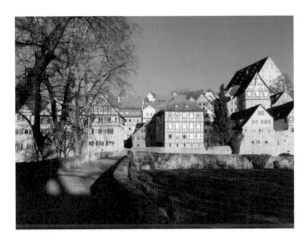

Walk to school in Schwaebisch Hall

My parents worked in Schwaebisch Hall at a general hospital known locally as *the Diak.* A Protestant order ran it. It was a safe haven from the privations of the War. Its grounds included residences for the sisters of the Order, a small nursing home for ailing retirees, residences for staff and a farm further up the river valley that guaranteed a basic food supply. A few mentally handicapped persons also lived on the grounds in a protected work arrangement. We lived in a converted medical ward in the main building of the hospital, my mom in pediatrics, my dad in internal medicine and radiology. During the War he was mostly at the Russian front and a complete stranger to me. I wet his knee when we first met. He shouldn't have put me there.

Fast-forward to the year of 1945. The Nazi regime was collapsing around our ears. The window of our dining room faced west, a fact of some significance, as allied bombers usually approached from there. We were having lunch. I sat at the side of the table that faced the window. A large formation of planes approached from the west with an increasing roar. I was transfixed by the sight and pointed at it. My parents did not share my delight. They grabbed me and fled to the bomb shelter in the basement of the hospital. A bomb hit with deafening crash. It shook everything. The reason for the commotion was a military airport located on a plain just above the hospital. German Messerschmitt 262 jet fighters were based there, and Allied Bomber Command had become interested. During one bombing run, an allied plane crashed into the hillside near the hospital. The crew's bodies may still rest there near an area that's now a burial place for the Sisters of the *Diakonissen Order*. Lots of truck-sized craters bore further witness to Bomber Command's efforts. Bombs hit the railway station and roads nearby. The historic old town remained untouched. It was like Russian roulette, with someone else pulling the trigger. One nearby town was wiped out entirely. After one bombardment my dad lifted me onto the sill for the view from our kitchen window. It overlooked the river valley below and the village of *Steinbach.* A bomb had hit a friend's house there. We had visited him just days before. It was ablaze like a huge torch. Days later, a nurse took me for a stroll outside during a lull in the fighting. Loud bangs and the stutter of machine guns chased us back inside. I felt curios and wasn't traumatized by any of this. My favorite memory of the War is about a small reconnaissance plane, probably a *Fieseler Storch.* It had belly-landed in a field near the airport. Maybe the pilot wanted to make a quick escape. Dad lifted me into the cockpit and I played with the controls, felt the plane shift under my seat when I moved a wing-flap and resolved instantly to become a pilot.

To me, war was harmless. Nothing bad would happen as long as my parents were with me. That sunny disposition didn't last. My mother died shortly after war's end of scarlet fever. No antibiotics were available to save her life. Her death changed everything at an age when bedtime stories and being tucked in still matter. A cold stepmother entered my life within the year and replaced warmth with maltreatment. I hid in a large closet amongst musty overcoats when the going got rough. I spent hours there, sometimes with a lit candle. I daydreamed a lot about being a great emperor and "commander" of a steam locomotive, a dual occupation that gave me the control I lacked elsewhere. Eventually dad surprised stepmother during one of our "disciplinary" sessions. He was forceful in my defense and it didn't happen again. Still my hackles rise whenever someone enjoys the exercise of power a bit too much. And mothballs still smell strangely reassuring.

We lived at the hospital for six more years after the war. I had the run of the place, stirred soups in the hospital kitchen in giant electrical kettles and developed advanced skills as a food taster. I became a connoisseur of cheese sandwiches and ate more strawberries than I cleaned in my role of kitchen helper. The night watchman's St. Bernard dog let me ride on its wide back and towed my toy cart. My father's motorcar was equally accommodating. It responded to a push of the starter button without a key, moving back and forth when a gear was engaged. This depleted the battery and the garage was declared off limits. A visit to the septic laundry resulted in a scrub-down with an antiseptic and a caution, sneaking into the operating room during a surgical procedure in a swift eviction. I got my very first Hershey bar off a black GI by staring at it until he forked it over. I also snuck into the hospital morgue with one of my little friends. A dead motorcyclist lay there on a gurney with his boots sticking out from under a sheet. The room was only half-lit by opaque windows and eerily quiet. A strange smell pervaded it. That was enough for the two of us. We turned tail and ran. Back home, our maid added a dose of folklore to the fright. The motorcyclist might have been a "non-dead," the kind that sits up suddenly and gets nasty. I swallowed her tale hook, line and sinker and got really scared of dead bodies, not what you want for a medical career. But I built a solid base for one in other ways.

We lived on a converted ward just a few floors below the radiology department for the first ten years of my life. The arrangement kept my dad available for emergencies at a moment's notice. His mornings never varied. First he put on dark-red goggles to prepare his eyes for a radiology screen that produced only faint images. Then he had a smoke, downed the dregs of his coffee, put on a white lab coat and took the elevator a few floors up to the radiology department. Once there, he donned a lead apron that must have weighted many pounds, insufficient protection though against the ambient radiation of his x-ray equipment. (Years of exposure gave him a low white blood count.) I joined him behind the screen in the darkness of the radiology room, equally protected. His patients didn't seem to mind the child radiologist. And I was thrilled to see a barium swallow slide down an esophagus, discover fractures, gallstones and gastric ulcers highlighted against a dark background by the contrast medium.

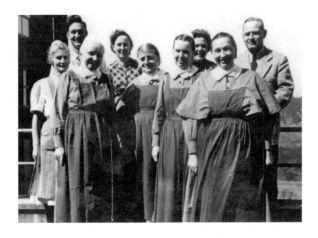

Dad (top right) and his radiology crew

Doctors were in short supply after the War. In addition to radiology, dad moonlighted in family practice and home visits. Most visits were for minor ailments. Once I accompanied him to the bedside of a man gravely ill with ascites, the fluid that accumulates in the abdomen during liver failure. We came to a dismal-looking little house. The patient was in bed in a cold room. Dad lit the wood stove and waited for the room to warm, then drained the ascites from the man's distended abdomen into a bucket through a large-bore needle. This may have been primitive, but reducing the pressure in his abdomen eased his breathing. There was no question of payment on this occasion. Other home visits were more remunerative. Most paid in kind. Large farms were the best. They provided us with eggs, milk, hunks of pork and poultry. Some served hot meals, pig's knuckles in kraut and other hearty stuff. The arrangement benefited both parties. Dad was the farmers' main source of healthcare, and they were an important source of food for us. The visits forged lasting bonds. Farmers consulted him for years about their woes whenever they caught him hunting out on the fields, and he always lent a patient ear. One provided Christmas turkeys for years after we had moved to a house in town. The beasts wouldn't fit into our small oven there. But the nuns helped out and roasted the beasts in the cavernous hospital oven. I took care to balance the casserole in the back of the car on the way home, making sure that the turkey tasted ok. - Say "turkey" now and I'll salivate like one of Pavlov's dogs.

My old man had some classy connections. One was a real live Count, the *Goetz of Berlchingen*. He lived in a 16th century chateau with surrounding moat and large grounds. His son was about my age. He took me to the stables and through stately rooms with tall gothic windows, vaulted ceilings and many artifacts, now part hotel and part museum. I got to touch the famous "Iron Hand" from the Sixteen Hundreds, a prosthetic device used by an ancestor after his forearm had been chopped off in the 1504 battle of Landshut. Riding the scooter of the young "Goetz" was another treat. Its balloon tires made for a cushy ride and saddled me a lasting preference for the life of the other half.

But it was the pig that really took the biscuit.

Food was rationed after the War. All live pigs were registered. Slaughter required a permit, but there was a loophole. There always is. The existence of a pig was registered, but not its size. This small omission enabled a lively black market, and my old man was in on it. When a sow had piglets, one of them could be exchanged for a mature pig that was ready for slaughter. Years' later dad filled me in over a glass of wine on the story and my role as a cover for the enterprise. We set out in a black two-stroke pre-War vintage DKW (*Deutscher KraftWagen*) that the occupying "*Amis*" (Americans) had licensed for medical practice. This time we weren't visiting a sickbed. We visited a farmyard and picked up a big fat pig. It was uncooperative at first and squealed when stuffed into the back of the DKW. But it kept quiet under a blanket for as long as the engine was running. On the way home we came to a military roadblock. Dad slowed the car, but kept the engine running. The soldiers knew him, had a look at innocent little me in the front seat and waved us through. Back at the hospital he retrieved his (illegal) service pistol from a hiding place behind a high-voltage sign in Radiology and shot the pig. The night was spent butchering, frying, bottling and canning the various bits and pieces, this after everyone within smelling range had been bribed to keep mum.

Grammar school (*Volksschule*) lacked psychological subtleties. It drilled us in the basics of reading, writing and math through exercises that we repeated over and over again, out loud and in chorus until the lesson stuck. Teachers pulled hair and ears to improve attention spans. Minor disciplinary infractions earned whacks with a bamboo cane on palms and fingers. This was called a "paw" and stung badly. If you had been really bad, a more thorough caning was scheduled for the following day, delayed to give the perpetrator time to think about it. On the day of reckoning the class waited in complete silence. Two boys seated behind a front-row desk held the perpetrator by his arms as he lay across their desk, presenting his derriere to the rod. Everybody watched for the sake of betterment. Experienced perps put on *Lederhosen* stuffed with newspaper, to prevent red welts and the need to explain these to their parents. They also yelped convincingly, in keeping with our Eleventh and Twelfth Commandments of "don't get caught" and "always fight back."

Religious instruction was mandatory in our curriculum, probably as an antidote to atheist Nazi ideology. Schwaebisch Hall was proud of its historical role during the Reformation. Martin Luther had sat under an ancient oak tree that still stands a few miles west of town. The reformer Johannes Brenz still is a household name. And all my friends were Protestant. Naturally, I joined them for religious instruction, no questions asked. A few months later, my emerging Lutheran fervor alerted my catholic parents. They asked questions and had me shifted over to their side. - *Cuius regio, cuius religio.* (Whoever rules, determines your religion; from the Europe's Wars over Religion.)

Religion hadn't done much to prevent Nazism. But it increased our food supply. American Quakers donated school lunches after the War, stodgy soups brewed locally and ladled into dented aluminum pots that did second duty as footballs. We weren't spoilt, but we didn't go hungry. Fridays brought a hint of carnal joy with chocolate milk in large containers and piles of sweet soft buns.

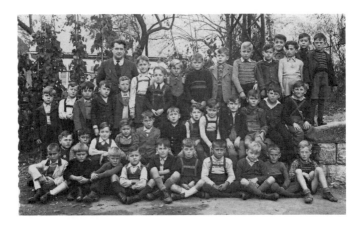

Grammar school; the author is the last one on the left, second row up, next to a future Lufthansa flight engineer looking equally grim.

Gymnasium (high school) opened the door to higher learning. It emphasized humanitarian ideals over piety and was seriously highbrow. Antiquity occupied center stage. Latin was taught from day one and for the entire nine years of the curriculum. We became closely acquainted with Greek Gods and the Roman emperors, read Julius Caesar's *"De Bello Gallico,"* Seneca's speeches and Ovid's poems, all in the original. Philosophy was an integral part of the curriculum. We studied Kant and Humboldt. (Don't ask for quotes.) My dad introduced me to Nietzsche. The natural sciences were both mandatory and entertaining. Given half a chance, we'd use laboratory equipment to make things stink and go "bang." I brought home a small bag of red phosphorus and an oxidant, then made the mistake of combining both. I was lucky. The resulting bang was loud enough to alarm the entire house, the damage limited to a tattered lampshade. History lessons were more cautious than chemistry. They stopped at WWII. Hitler happened, but you had to ask for details. Fortunately, a catholic minister filled us in with filmed evidence of the holocaust. English and French were afterthoughts, taught only briefly towards the end of the 9-year curriculum. I learned to converse in Latin but not in any modern language. Music lessons began with Johann Sebastian Bach, moved on to Mozart and Beethoven and stayed there. We sang Latin corals, me off-tune to get out of choral duty. Pop was frowned upon and considered coarse. I didn't listen to the Beatles until medical school. Psychology wasn't taught at all, and I finished school without any idea about what made me tick.

The Gymnasium may look antiquated in hindsight. But it had its advantages. It relied only rarely on rote learning, encouraged curiosity, skepticism and debate.

Besides making things smoke, stink and go "bang," hunting and fishing were my favorite pastimes. They were more than that. They were a way of life. I spent countless hours in the woods, on tree stands and by the river at dan and dusk, watching deer emerge cautiously from the edge of the woods onto the meadows, an owl perching on a branch right next to me and a deer giving birth. I slept in a hammock high up in trees to be at the right spot at dawn for a boar, this until my hammock broke one night and I woke up on the ground with a very sore head. I spend long evenings on the bank of our slow-moving river, waiting for my fishing rod to bend as an eel took the bait. I waited amongst the reeds for squawking flights of ducks and listened to hares bouncing through the dead leaves in fall, appearing at long last as a shadow at the edge of the field. When nothing was going on, I read books until darkness fell. During the summer holidays I trolled for trout and pike with my Bavarian uncle in the *Forggensee*, a lake below *Neuschwanstein Castle* of King Ludwig fame. In fall, I joined the local hunt with my dad, an activity that involved more eating, drinking and singing in pubs than time in misty woods. – I was determined to stick with the only life that seemed worth living.

Medical school was a natural choice for someone who had grown up in a hospital and had several doctors in the family. I volunteered out of curiosity when a school psychologist offered free aptitude testing. To everyone's surprise he suggested law, not medicine as my natural field of study. To see what this was like, I joined my uncle in Fuessen, a small town in Southern Bavaria. Fuessen sits astride a medieval trade route that meanders south from the North Sea through the length of Germany, from there across the Alps and all the way down into Italy. White *Neuschwanstein Castle* stands out nearby against a dark alpine backdrop. A medieval castle dominates the old town. It housed the courtroom.

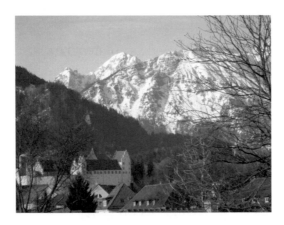

Fuessen Castle

My uncle was Fuessen's government veterinarian and meat inspector, testifying in a legal case over the quality of sausage casings. Sausages, especially the white variety, are to Bavarians what mothers' milk is to babies. My uncle was a genuine local. He owned an impressive red moustache and a big nose he would touch with his tongue, if you asked nicely. In court, he wore green Loden cloth and fended off lawyers' questions in dialect with a wicked sense of humor. Non-Bavarians would have needed subtitles. The judge learned all there was to know about the differences between fake and natural gut for sausage casings and why this mattered. I loved the occasion, but not the drawn-out proceedings and ignored the psychologist's advice. Many years later fate would take me to the Courts of Law anyway. Maybe the psychologist knew something after all.

Psychiatry also wasn't on my radar screen. Even further from my mind was work on "funny farms," the large psychiatric institutions that sheltered the incurably insane until antipsychotic medications rendered them obsolete. One day, a visit to a "farm" near Lake Konstanz was on my dad's agenda. He was visiting his ward, a woman doctor who had been declared permanently incompetent for reason of insanity. (Thankfully, a finding of incompetence can nowadays be challenged.) Why not have a look? We set out in his gray Mercedes Benz, he in his gray suit, gray tie and white shirt, understated as always. The landscape around Lake Konstanz is gorgeous, with mature woods, rolling hills, vineyards and small winding roads. A nearby cluster of Romanesque churches goes back to the tenth century. - It's now a World Heritage site. - We drove along a tree-lined alee to a grand old house in a park-like setting. Dad went inside to confer with his ward, and I explored the grounds. His ward accompanied him outside as he was leaving. He introduced us. She was painfully shy, barely looked me in the eye and became tearful when saying goodbye. Dad promised another visit soon. He must have been her main link to the outside world.

Brother Kuch

German medical school weeds out the faint and the nauseous by requiring two month's work as a hospital orderly. I served my time at the *Diak*, the place where I was born, where I had lived for the first ten years of my life, where my mother had died and where my dad would die just months before my graduation. "Brother Kuch" was my handle. He didn't get a special deal. At 6 a.m. he layered three aprons carefully over a long monkish gown for the first task of the day, emptying bedpans and urine flasks. He then cleaned the lot, washed bums, made beds, collected greenish gobs of sputum for the lab and distributed chamomile tea to patients from a trolley down a linoleum hallway. (I still abhor chamomile smell and linoleum hallways.) Afterwards he sat down at a long table together with other orderlies, said Grace and demolished a sustaining breakfast of pork cutlets, sausages, potatoes and more chamomile tea. When called to pick up an *"exitus"* (a dead body or "stiff"), the two orderlies who had drawn the short straw would grab a covered gurney, taking care to arrive when nobody was looking. The corpse was usually in a small room darkened by curtains drawn. They would lift it onto the gurney, wheel it to the service elevator and out onto the street. From there it was a short run down a hill and to the morgue, a small building shaded by large trees (the site of my earlier encounter with the "non-dead" motor cyclist). We always covered the distance in a hurry and rarely encountered anyone. A gallows' humor prevailed amongst orderlies and patients alike on these occasions. Patients consoled us despite the fact that they too might occupy similar transport, and we knocked back a schnapps, curtesy of a kindly innkeeper who had an enlarged liver for a reason and a sizeable stash in his locker.

Most patients were local farmers, hearty but gruff and not overly clean. We scrubbed them after admission until they glistened. According to a standing joke, both feet needed cleaning, not just the afflicted one before the doctor would see you. After a week or two on the ward many also needed "emptying out." The hospital diet was high in starch and fat and low in fiber. Immobility did the rest. Requests for laxatives were routine, enemas a sought-after remedy. An old hand in these matters introduced Brother Kuch to a concoction that was easily administered rectally and fabulously effective. It contained warm glycerin, a pinch of salt and a secret ingredient for added potency. Once injected into the victim's derriere, his face would assume a puzzled expression that quickly changed to urgency. Fame grew with each spectacular result. - I could have opened a practice in gastroenterology right then and there.

Heidelberg Medical School

Ruperta Carola is the name of Heidelberg University and the home of the "Student Prince." *Gaudeamus igitur* (lets have fun) goes the famous student song, and I intended to do just that. My new life began at a lads-only residence located in Schriesheim, a village outside Heidelberg nestled beneath vineyards and a ruined chateau, the *Strahlenburg*. Disrespectful locals nicknamed it the "bulls' cloister." It was the perfect place for male bonding, and I made life-long friends there. We drank local wine and sang student songs from the pages of a *"beer bible"* with studs on its hardcover, that kept it dry from spilled beer. We listened to Beethoven, Schubert and Wagner, seven or eight of us crammed into a small bed-sitter, and cooked blistering-hot curries in the communal kitchen with spices provided by a student from Malaysia, finally free from adult supervision. Pranks were obligatory. J, the owner of the residence, was a natural target of juvenile rebellion. He operated a distillery next door that produced a schnapps labeled *"Hochspannung"* (high voltage). It guaranteed a rowdy party and a monumental headache the morning after. A few of us swore off hard liquor for life. Besides being a merchant of inebriation, J also was a man of faith. We provoked his religious side by quoting Nietzsche's "God is dead." He in turn did all he could to prove that God's is still alive, reminding us that "not even the Heidelberg tram can operate without a *Fuehrer* (leader). How then can the world?" Women were banned from the "bulls' cloister" between dusk and dawn, but enforcement was a dismal failure. Decrees drawn up in elaborate Gothic script declared our unalienable right to agnostic liberty and carnal happiness. One student produced *Berger* charges, a combustible mix used in WWII to fog in tank positions, effective also against hapless farmers plowing their fields. We joined street demonstrations in support of progressive causes. Baptism by water cannon became a rite of passage. And then, when we were in full flight, two of our mates broke ranks and joined a rightwing dueling fraternity. Its members are easily recognizable even nowadays by scars on the lower left side of their faces, proof positive of manliness achieved by wounding in a rapier duel. Their fraternity hats resembled those of baggage carriers at the railway station, evoking unflattering comparisons. But we still drank and sang together. A nighttime visit at Heidelberg Castle led to a mock sword fight amid ancient walls. One medical student, now a respected prof, won a suckling pig at a wine festival raffle. It survived as a mascot in the music room until administration threatened eviction. The difference between now and then in the life of medical students is striking. Today's students learn more medicine than we did. We learned more about having fun. Attendance checks were rare. We slept in, read novels and travelled to nearby France. Conviviality mattered more than anything else to a bunch of kids who had come straight from the bosom of the family. I learned this the hard way after moving to a one-bedroom rental in downtown Heidelberg. My room was in the old part of town, near the Castle and many pubs. It had a ceramic stove, high ceilings and looked romantic. The reality wasn't. It was miles from the "bulls' cloister." There was nobody around to talk to or cook with. Cellphones and social media were decades away and dropping in for a visit rarely worked. After one semester on my own I moved back into another student residence, this one closer to downtown. The *"Klausenpfad"* is still there.

Our teaching facilities were Spartan. Medical students attended lectures on chemistry and physics together with the "real" physicists and chemists. The lecture halls were far too small for that. Only the highly motivated managed to pile in, and I wasn't one of them. Anatomy was never overcrowded though, and for a good reason. An inscription over its classicist portal gave a hint: *"Hic Gaudet Mors Succurrere Vitae."* (Here It Pleases Death To Assist The Living.) Corpses awaited dissection there and anything exposed to them smelled rancid and of formaldehyde, tools, clothes and medical student. A morning spent at Anatomy was enough to clear squeamish art students from a table at the *Mensa* (the student cafeteria). I spent an entire week there, patiently dissecting a hand and learning a great many Latin terms, but not why that mattered. Physiology was less smelly. It also made more sense. It offered a first description of the **feedback loops** that control self-regulating organisms (including human behavior, as shown later). Disorders like diabetes and hyperthyroidism develop when feedback loops go awry. Pharmacology took us back to learning by rote. We learned how to distill heart medication from digitalis plants and make toothpaste from scratch. I recited a collection of one hundred prescriptions daily from index cards until the morning of the exam. - I have never used even one.

Over the course of two years, our student cohort dwindled by half. Getting into medical school had been easy. Tuition was (and still is) free of charge and anyone with a high school diploma could get in. Senseless cramming weeded out anyone lacking in frustration tolerance. Examiners tossed out a few more who weren't thinking on their feet. The anatomy prof showed me a microscopic cut of tissue with a mucous membrane on one side and a hairy epidermis on the other. Thick hairs were rooted in small vesicles, an unusual sight and not a part of any anatomy lesson. I confessed my ignorance, then described in detail what I saw. He explained that it was from a cat's lip, and passed me.

Passing basic science exams opened the door to the clinical part of medical school, the part that would turn us into doctors. Close contact with live patients remained limited and offered no room for initiative. Lecturers went from hospital bed to hospital bed during visitations, hands clasped behind backs, us following behind like chicks behind mother goose. I felt uninspired and decamped to Munich for a bit of fun. There a budgetary inconvenience developed. To remedy this, I took a job in Shipping and Receiving at a suburban loo paper factory and turned myself into a workingman in overalls and heavy boots. It was a brave new world. The factory-made toilet rolls in white, pink and blue. We punched in at eight in the morning and packaged "bog rolls" (loo paper rolls) as rapidly as possible. I leaned to fold sharp creases for perfectly squared packages and made sure that the correct color went to the correct village. Occasionally the factory owner checked on our productivity, to be regarded with sideways glances and socialist hostility. Around ten o'clock our crew went to the pub across the street for a liter or two of Munich brew. Lunchtime brought more beer. We quit around five, memory being a bit hazy by then. Evenings were a dead loss. I felt too tired for anything beyond a meal at a pub. The excitement of being a workingman faded. Financial health restored, Shipping and Receiving looked like a rut and medical school looked better by the day. A job offer of night watchman failed to convince, even after an Alsatian dog was thrown in as a hiring bonus.

Back in Heidelberg came the time to choose a topic for a doctorate, the German *"Dr. med."* The doctorate was optional, but my parents had it and so would I. Pathology looked like the very embodiment of scientific medicine. I preferred it to the hustle and bustle of clinical care. Wilhelm Doerr was my role model. He was Heidelberg's Chair in Pathology, a brilliant lecturer, author of many research papers and a voluminous textbook. I applied, and he appointed me to a satellite institute in Karlsruhe less than an hour's drive from Heidelberg. My job included conducting autopsies and studying a recently discovered cell type in the horse pancreas, this in the hope of restoring insulin-production in diabetics. The latter was my doctoral thesis.

The Karlsruhe Institute had the imperial looks of a traditional North American bank. It was built for eternity. Greek columns fronted a grand entrance hall. Twelve-foot ceilings, tall windows and neo-baroque ornaments made for an imposing interior. Its wood-paneled library was a temple of knowledge, its floor-to-ceiling bookshelves crammed with textbooks and journals. The sweet smell of dead bodies permeated everything. It was the perfect place to confront my fear of dead bodies. The morgue was in the basement, hidden from prying eyes. Its huge stainless-steel refrigerator held some 20 gurneys on rollers that functioned like drawers in a cupboard. Corpses waited there for their appointment with the pathologist, some still in street clothing and looking freakishly life-like. The adjacent autopsy room was the size of a small lecture hall. It housed four steel slabs equipped with running water and drains. No sounds from the outside world penetrated there, and everything was kept meticulously clean. Here I would wield knife and saw on the dead, to find out what might have gone wrong with their care.

Read on at your own risk.

Cutting into human flesh evokes ancient reflexes, even if you don't believe in the "non-dead." Their only response to deep cuts was passive movement. We explored every nook and cranny of their anatomy to leave no abnormality undetected. The first cut went from the base of the neck down to the pubes, deep enough to lay open the abdominal cavity. The abdominal wall was then retracted. Internal organs were laid bare for inspection. Heart, liver, guts and kidneys were removed and laid out on brown plastic trays for further examination. Next, a lateral cut split the skin around the dorsal base of the skull, forwards and upwards over the ears and downward again below the chin. This separated the face from the underlying bone and allowed it to be folded down over itself, freeing access to the skull. A circular saw opened the skull with a screeching noise. The brain was removed and examined. Seeing a corpse reduced within an hour from human being to faceless specimen is a startling lesson in mortality, one that still haunts me. Findings were conferenced with treating physicians standing around the opened corpse. The conference covered diagnosis, treatment and any errors that might have occurred. Never have I seen surgeons look more demure. After all was said and done, an orderly sewed the corpse back together, skillfully hiding cuts inside skin folds. The corpse looked dignified again for presentation to grieving relatives.

Normally relatives had to give their permission for an autopsy. This rule was waved for Court-ordered autopsies. Two Court-ordered autopsies proceeded in spite of passionate objections. During the first, relatives camped out on the doorstep of the Institute in protest. During the second, the local Daily fanned the flames of passion with a headline demanding to know "Who Owns Mother's Heart." A third Court-ordered autopsy proceeded without protest, but was controversial all the same. It had been arranged just before the funeral was to take place. The deceased had cut his son out of his will, and the son was contesting it. He claimed that his old man had been demented and therefor incapable of writing a valid will. The autopsy took place in the serene surroundings of a small funeral chapel, a scenario that could have been part of a horror movie. We snuck through the church yard and into the chapel through a side door, lifted the old man out of his casket where he had been laid out in his Sunday best and moved him onto a stretcher. There we sawed open his skull and removed the brain, bagged the lot and disappeared before the mourners arrived. The prof was scathing afterwards in his report: There was "no evidence whatsoever indicating dementia. The deceased had written his will during a lucid moment."

I survived my time at the Institute by sheer grit. Fear, nausea and faintness abated within weeks. Nightmares persisted. I lost weight and developed an aversion to meat and offal, augmented by the fact that local butchers displayed their wares on brown plastic trays identical to the ones we used for the display of human organs. Eventually I learned to view autopsies with "clinical" detachment, a vital skill in a line of work where most news is bad. A degree of clinical detachment is necessary in the practice of medicine. Too much of it is counter-productive. It transforms a living person who is "one of us" into a mere "specimen" studied without emotion. And that translates all too easily into an aloof bedside manner and a lack of empathy, not what distressed people need. It can also lead to a lack of caution. Whatever happens to the patient can also happen to the doctor, as I was soon to discover.

Close contact with dead bodies is risky. Precautions at the Karlsruhe Institute were basic. We used gloves, rubber aprons and rubber boots, but no facemasks or goggles. One orderly and one of the pathologists already suffered from tuberculosis (TB) when I started there. I did not wear a facemask when I removed the lungs from two victims of TB. I held them up by the trachea (windpipe), filled them with formaldehyde to solidify the tissue and sliced them, to demonstrate their tubercular lesions. Both corpses had lungs holed like Swiss cheese, indicative of severely contagious TB. Filling them with liquid displaced inside air and made TB germs airborne, a warning I received only after the fact. During a subsequent visit back home my dad noticed pallor, weight loss and night sweats, all potential symptoms of active TB. He put me in front of his x-ray screen, confirmed TB in its first stage and prescribed *tuberculostatics,* disregarding the usual rules of not treating family. His decisive intervention stopped the infection in its tracks, saved my health and my career. I recovered without a trace. It was a close call in several regards. TB can be fatal. It's also hard on surviving patients. In Sixties Germany, TB patients were quarantined in sanatoriums. Quarantine would have interrupted my studies or scuttled them entirely, as was the misfortune of a friend. I had to live cautiously for years after recovery, avoid excessive exertion and sun exposure, eat regularly, rest in the afternoons and go to bed early. It was quite a bore. I also had to keep my reasons for this restraint a secret, lest fear of TB from me might turn me into a pariah. A degree of social isolation was the unavoidable result. It was an object lesson on the **impact of an illness** beyond its physical symptoms, brilliantly illustrated by Thomas Mann's novel "The Magic Mountain." I almost took a second hit years later when I applied for immigrant status in Canada. Dutifully, I reported my complete medical history, then received notice that admission could not be granted. Luckily, a medical review board declared me fully recovered and safe to be around. And there was another lesson. Most medications have "side-effects," as did mine, albeit a pleasant one. One of my TB medications was the precursor of a modern antidepressant (a MAO inhibitor). It lifted my mood and turned shyness into extroversion. I felt reckless enough to embark on a summer at the University of Umea in Northern Sweden, never mind medical advice to the contrary and a complete lack of Swedish language skills. I am eternally glad though that I did, or I would have missed out on a transformative experience.

I hopped into my VW Beetle for the long drive north, through Denmark and most of the entire length of Sweden, on small roads, past a multitude of shimmering lakes, rocky shores and uninhabited forests. In Umea just below the Polar Circle, I joined a group of foreign exchange students, one from Communist Poland, one from Tito's Yugoslavia and a third from liberal Denmark. Together we enjoyed midnights bright enough to read the paper outdoors and a hospitality so generous, it was hard to believe. Smorgasbords, a midnight bonfire by the sea, outings far north of the polar circle, miles down into the bowels of a mine, to factories, a military installation, a cottage in Lapland and an overnight sailing trip were more than mere excursions. They were transformative, as was my stay at the university. I hadn't seen real wilderness before. I had never been welcomed like this before. Lectures were held in English to accommodate us visitors, and the Profs displayed a complete lack of hierarchical thinking. Access to teachers was easy, and medical care lacked bureaucracy. I never thanked my hosts properly, much to my regret.

A subsequent trip to the USSR contrasted starkly to liberal Sweden. I joined a university-sponsored group of six that traveled through several East-bloc countries and from there to Moscow, our main destination. The Cold War was at its height and tourists were thin on the ground. Memories from WWII were fresh. Access to Leningrad (now St. Petersburg) was denied for no apparent reason. We were objects of curiosity on the streets, regarded cautiously from afar. I still managed to go halves on a small bottle of vodka at the Gum department store and shared it on the spot. I tasted Beluga caviar for the first and probably last time in my life and coughed my way through a joint of Makhorka on a bus where a stranger paid for my ticket. I joined a long queue of socialist pilgrims in Red Square to visit a severe-looking Lenin in his glass coffin, rode the ornate subway that takes you deep underground and away from any bombs that might fall on Moscow. I managed to "lose" my KGB minder for an unscheduled outing to Zagorsk, a marvel of multi-domed churches and a lonely remnant of Orthodox services. The outing may have earned me an "invitation" from the KGP to the "House of Friendship," fortunately not the one at Dzerzhinsky Square, an offer I could not refuse. I turned up as ordered and was escorted to a large hall with cubicles that contained more uneasy-looking "friends." A man and a woman entered my cubicle, clad from head to toe in shiny black leather (standard KGB issue according to the KGB museum in Prague). I felt like a spy who hadn't made it home in time. The woman perched on the disk in front of me. She asked the questions in excellent German and translated for the senior-looking officer seated offside. He denied speaking German, but his reactions gave him away. Her questions made the desired answer perfectly clear. West German income taxes were progressive, I said. They were high for high earners, and poor people paid nothing. Medical school was free. This met with frowns, derisive smiles and more questions until

I got my answers right. Questions went from there to military installations I didn't know existed, to politics and German living conditions. I made things up as the hours passed, sounding as naïve and confused as I felt. Nobody laid a glove on me. I can't tell what the KGB expected to gain by interviewing me, except to confirm their particular worldview to themselves.

Back in a more relaxed Heidelberg, I typed my doctoral dissertation with carbon copies for backup and devoted its slim volume to my father shortly before his death. The doctorate dealt with "bright cells" in the pancreatic ducts of the horse, not exactly a household topic. The cells were thought to be potential insulin-producers, this according a Viennese pathologist named Feyeter. Examining them under a fluoroscope was painstaking work. Photographs had to be taken in the middle of the night. Exposure times lasted hours, to avoid tremors from passing streetcars that might disrupt the stillness of the image. My research was later quoted in a textbook on the pancreas, shockingly without attribution. Chairman Doerr intervened and my labors appeared in the German Journal of Gastroenterology, an unusual distinction for a medical student. They surfaced once again decades later in Google Books. By then new research had dashed any hopes for a treatment of diabetes by cultivating "bright cells." - The cells produce heparin, not insulin.

Preparations for the final Medical Boards consumed my attention in the months following my father's death. Board exams were exclusively oral and taken jointly by groups of four candidates. Assembling a smart group was vitally important. One underperformer could spoil the team effort. We studied together and soaked our brains in caffeine before exams. Internal medicine, surgery, pathology, infectious diseases, pharmacology, neurology and psychiatry were all packed into just a few months. A pressure cooker atmosphere resulted, that gave recurrent nightmares to many graduates. Mine lasted for years and were always the same: Exams are approaching and a mountain of mandatory reading must be mastered in an impossibly brief period of time. One member of our group went without sleep for days, then froze during an oral exam and flunked. I passed all subjects, with one career-changing hiccup. My psychiatric case was a middle-aged woman who had no complaints whatsoever, not even about being an involuntary patient in a locked ward with windows barred. She was cheerful, difficult to interrupt and tried to sell me a stamp collection. This should have set off several alarms, but I didn't know what to look for. I missed her diagnosis of hypomania and returned a verdict of obsessive-compulsive disorder (OCD), a special interest of my examiner Dr. Tellenbach. This failed to please. His face grew stern and I feared the worst. Flunking psychiatry with a "5" would have nixed my entire board exam and have me start up all over again. Instead of lowering the hammer, he extracted a promise: I must include a rotation in psychiatry with my internship. If I gave my word of honor, he would give me a "4", a bare pass. I did and he did.

Defending my doctoral thesis was a walk in the park by comparison. I was a doctor now, or so I thought. I knew lots of theory and little about practice. I was a blank sheet, determined to explore whatever was of interest.

Internship

In the Sixties Germany required two years of rotating internships before issuing a general license to practice medicine. This was a very good idea. Most graduates had yet to learn how to lay sutures, set bones, perform minor operations, deliver babies and write appropriate prescriptions. We would learn on the job during three obligatory six-month rotations in internal medicine, surgery, obstetrics and gynecology. The fourth six-month rotation would fulfill my (unenforceable) promise to upgrade my knowledge in psychiatry. I wasn't prepared to work on Dr. Tellenbach's locked ward at the university hospital, and applied at the Max Planck Institute for Psychiatric Research in Heidelberg with the confidence of youth. My interviewer there, a former Olympian, ignored excellent graduation scores in all subjects except psychiatry, noted mediocre high school grades and recommended "foreign experience" as a primer for any work at the Institute. I parked this for later use and moved to Starnberg, a picturesque town on a lake just south of Munich. The manic-depressive King Ludwig of Bavaria had drowned himself there, not a good omen for a future psychiatrist. The first available position was in **pediatrics** at the general hospital. I started work on a ward for immature newborns, moved from there to an isolation ward for children with infectious diseases and then to a ward for children with allergies and asthma.

Some newborns were admitted in the middle of the night in a state of life-threatening dehydration. A nurse would prepare the necessary paraphernalia and immobilize the screaming baby. The intern on night call would wipe the sleep out of his eyes and settle down on a stool besides the crib, to perform the fiddly task. Usually, no veins could be located in the baby's arms. Instead, a tiny butterfly needle had to be inserted into an equally tiny vein in the baby's scalp, quite a challenge for someone who had never done anything like this before. The screaming helped, as it made the veins bulge. Rehydration was essential to the baby's survival and failure was not an option. Sleep was impossible afterwards. Much could have gone wrong and, when it did, grief-stricken parents had to be informed. The kids on the isolation ward were healthier by comparison, once they were past the feverish stage. They still weren't allowed to receive visitors though. They needed company and laughs, an invitation to all kinds of monkey business. One game involved an outdated psychological test. The child is asked to draw her family as animals. Results can be revealing. One dad was portrayed as a "hippo" looming large above the others. A grandmother was an "alligator" with wide-open jaws, ready to take on cowering relations. It was fun, and I felt tempted to stay. Some kids called me "daddy" though, a role I wasn't ready for. Some asthmatic kids recovered quickly upon admission and relapsed just as quickly after discharge. A psychiatric consultation might have been in order there. Senior staff was supportive and never talked down to us interns, as seemed customary later on at the downtown Munich hospitals where I worked next.

The **surgery** rotation at a small private hospital in a fancy suburb was excellent for hands-on practice, but it lacked supervision. I laid my very first suture to a girl's forehead during night call entirely on my own. Luckily, no scarring developed afterwards on follow-up. I assisted with abdominal surgeries and removed an inflamed appendix with the sole assistance of an experienced OR nurse. I intubated (inserted airways) and ventilated patients in my role of neo-anesthesiologist, monitored vital signs and coped with sudden drops in blood pressure. Applying plaster casts to fractures became routine, with one hiccup. I was blamed for a poorly healing fracture I had not set. My relationship with nurses and junior staff was close. With the chief surgeon and clinic owner it was as distant as I could make it.

An equally small private hospital for **obstetrics and gynecology** was next. It offered even less supervision than the surgery rotation. At one point the chief went abroad on holiday and the sole resident physician took ill. I was left to deliver a stillborn on my own, without back up. Fortunately, my patient's spouse was a physician. He was calmer than I felt and a capable assistant, and the delivery went without a hitch. I also ran the outpatient clinic for an entire week, prescribed colorful but useless vitamin injections and accelerated return visits. When the chief finally returned, I complained. He offering an apple from his garden as a "reward," knowing full well that gynecology rotations were hard to find in Munich. He looked surprised when I quit on the spot. - His conduct would attract censure nowadays. Back then, chief physicians were like gods, and some behaved accordingly.

An acquaintance helped me find a job at the university hospital, to complete the gynecology requirement for certification. I worked there without pay, attending dying women on a cancer ward. The "cottage" occupied a small open-plan building besides the main facility. It offered little privacy for its patients beyond curtains. Few were discharged alive. Most died silently, sedated by generous doses of morphine. We had an "open pharmacy" arrangement. Nuns with flowery names like "Rose" and "Hyacinth" administered whatever was required for pain relief. Some patients had radioactive inserts for the palliative reduction of uterine tumors. Lead aprons for radiation protection were in short supply. We went on some of our daily rounds with a nun positioned between junior doctor and radioactive patient, to shield our valuable fertility.

My last rotation was in **cardiology** at another university hospital. I was responsible for a large room with a dozen patients in varying stages of cardiac failure. They were incurable by any means available then, anxious for news and waiting patiently for a life-saving intervention that never came. We made the rounds every morning, offered reassurance and then moved on without detailed discussions about prognosis. Fortunately, visits from friends and relatives were ample and the patients had each other for company. Still, it was a depressing sight. A brief stint on a dermatology ward offered some diversion. There my job included inspecting rashes and recording their progress over time by marking a blank body silhouette with the areas affected by the rash.

I felt vastly relieved by the end of my rotating internship. I was licensed to practice general medicine now, with one large fly in the ointment. I felt doubtful about my professional future. There had to be something more positive than my internship and something less dangerous to my health than pathology. What could that be? Luck and a solid dose of chutzpah helped with the next step. I had studied from American textbooks for my boards. With their help and no particular goal in mind, I took yet another exam, this one at *Ramstein* US Air Force Base near Frankfurt. - Passing the ECFMG (Educational Council for Foreign Medical Graduates) would qualify me to work in US medical facilities. Why not try for it and see what happens?

Once on the base I was herded to a barren-looking classroom together with some twenty other foreign-looking candidates. We sat down at widely-spaced school desks and received sheets with multiple-choice questions. These we completed in total silence while suspicious military police marched up and down the aisle, making damned sure those foreigners didn't cheat. I passed, and qualified for further training at an accredited American hospital. I also took a lengthy psychological test (the MMPI) at the request of a potential employer that didn't want to import a freak or psychopath. My MMPI box ticking must have looked acceptably flat, and another door opened. A US military base in Lyon looked like the best of all choices. Located in Southern France, it combined American training with French ambience and the company of locals I had met through my dad. I went there to apply. Then politics intervened. De Gaulle quit NATO and the Lyon base closed. In for a penny, in for a pound. I wasn't backing off now and looked for a job across the pond.

Sweden's openness had been great. The USA was Sweden on steroids. A brief enquiry yielded multiple job offers, amongst them a surgery residency in Hawaii, a neuropathology residency in Chicago, an internship in New Jersey and two psychiatry residencies, one in New York and another one in Florida. All but one were university positions, to me an essential qualifier. Which one should I choose, having no particular career plans and knowing next to nothing about the USA? Going back into pathology felt too risky for health reasons. Surgery in Hawaii looked glamorous, but was too far from home. New York sounded overwhelming. The University of Florida was in a small town, promised a sub-tropical experience, and its name evoked floral imagery. I made a beeline for it, listened to *"Luncheon In Munchen"* on the American Forces Network in preparation and took an English course at an interpreters' school. I flunked the course, but never mind. One year in Florida would release me from my pledge of a rotation in psychiatry, get me fluent in English and administer a dose of American training. Thereafter, opportunities in Germany would be plentiful, or so I thought. I hopped on a flight to the Big Apple in October of 1968 with plans to travel south to Florida by road.

New York introduced me to "Hair" the musical, to skyscrapers, a startling degree of social directness and the importance of just going for it. A glamorous PANAM stewardess of local acquaintance (sorry, no romance) coached me in the essentials: "Speak up. Don't hide your light under a bushel. Sound enterprising. And smile a lot." I tried to buy a used Ford Mustang convertible but lacked the necessary credit. Then an elderly New Yorker placed an ad in the New York Times to have his car transferred to his winter residence near Miami. What better way to go south than with his wheels while taking in the sights? After passing an eye exam and answering a few questions posed by the owner's agency, I went to a large parking garage in Manhattan to retrieve his car. It was an enormous Cadillac, fully automatic, air-conditioned and with power brakes that could catapult a novice through the windshield. It started on first try, and off I went without hitting anything. That was the good news. Manhattan had absolutely no road signs pointing towards "Miami, Florida." After half a day of aimless driving I discovered the value of road maps, but not how much time the trip was going to take. I decided on the scenic costal route instead of the Interstate, drove and drove through towns big and small, stopped over in Washington and continued along swamps and through forests with increasingly unfamiliar vegetation. I exchanged wool for cotton as I entered the Deep South, shed layer after layer and developed a deepening appreciation for air-conditioning. I learned to say "hi, fill'er up" and "how are 'ya." The owner of the caddy was not amused by my late arrival. The university was more forgiving.

Gainesville was indeed a small town. (It is no more.) I exited the highway, drove down Main Street, took a few turns and found myself back in the countryside. I had wanted something completely different, and I got it in spades. To the European eye Florida is vast. Cities with palm-fringed multi-lane avenues, long empty coastal roads, flyblown swamps with alligators lurking in the weeds, Spanish moss floating from oaks and cypress trees, solitude and settlers' grit left deep impressions. I barely spoke enough English to make basic conversation, not enough to make friends. It was tough. And then, gradually, something happened. The place grew on me, sunsets over the Gulf of Mexico, vast empty beaches, dunes of warm white sand, rustic bars, fried catfish and oysters, whiskey sours, rocking chairs on wooden porches and good ole' boys' humor. Gospel singing to a beat-up piano and rhythmic stomping by the faithful that made a small whitewashed Baptist church rock on its stilts. It was more than unforgettable. The South imprinted itself on me.

One experience was straight out of the movies. I was driving an old convertible along the coastal road near Cedar Key, then a small fishing village where houses sat on stilts in the still waters of the Gulf of Mexico. The setting sun cast a golden glow. A lean man in jeans was relaxing on a porch, his Stetson pushed back onto the back of his head. His boots rested on the bannister. He was having a smoke, the very image of cool. I parked at a respectful distance and put up my boots as well in the back of the convertible. It was so quiet "you could hear a chicken sneeze," as Woody Guthrie put it in a song. And then, far away, I heard the wail of a police siren. It drew nearer. The man didn't move. The cruiser came to a screeching halt in front of the little house. Two cops jumped out, grabbed their man and dumped him into the back of the cruiser. Doors slammed. The cruiser started up, kicking gravel. And the wail of the siren faded slowly in the distance, silence renewed.

The image seems emblematic of the times. There was beauty in it, a hint of ease and adventure, with trouble lurking just beneath the surface. The late Sixties were a time of growing affluence, of blues, jazz and country music, Woodstock, a divisive Vietnam War with far too many casualties and protests spreading nation-wide. Florida changed and it changed me while acquainting me with American psychiatry.

2.WHICH END IS UP?

My first assignment in Gainesville was on a psychiatric ward at the Veterans' Administration Hospital. Security vetting was mandatory, including a two-page list of communist associations I had never heard of. I swore I wasn't a member of any of them, got my nametag and was introduced to the staff on the psychiatric inpatient unit.

Any new job requires an adjustment. This one was huge, to the point of being disorienting. I was new to the country, its climate and its way of life. My English was poor and Southern slang almost unintelligible. The banter and teasing that Southerners dish out to people they like came across like subtle insults. I felt defensive, knew little about the military and had never dealt with army veterans before. I was unfamiliar with American prescription drugs and had to look up most of them, their indications, doses and side effects. I was painfully slow. A stiff upper lip helped. Friendly nurses, fellow residents and my supervisor helped a lot more. I got used to redneck humor, but never quite managed a Southern drawl. An English lady, daughter of a member in the House of Lords, tried to save me from going native by teaching me "proper English." Whereupon a local called me "a goddamn Yankee." I must have looked taciturn through much of this with my fear of causing offense. My first supervisor was Henry Lyons. He was an Air Force veteran, tall, lanky, with sharp creases in his pants and sporting a regulation crew cut. He parked his boots on his desk when in relaxed mode, which was often, steadied me with his dry wit and easygoing manner. Nothing seemed to unsettle him. He wasn't all medicine either, took me fishing in the Gulf of Mexico where we caught grouper, snapper, sea trout and catfish and offered a tongue-in-cheek introduction to the countryside around Gainesville: "Kuch," he cautioned, "if you see a black-faced snake (a poisonous moccasin), don't pick it up." He was exactly what I needed.

There was more to lighten the mood on a ward dedicated to relieving distress and misery. One of the nurses was mortally afraid of snakes. She also liked fishing in a nearby lake, and, being a plucky lady, she carried a six-shooter when venturing there, just in case. Which is how she acquired her reputation as a fast draw. She was drifting peacefully under Cyprus trees, bathing her worm, when a snake dropped from a tree into her dingy. Startled, she emptied her six-shooter in its direction. Its caliber was large and it holed her boat close to sinking.

Most veterans admitted to our ward had returned recently from 'Nam, a place not known for its benign environment. They were edgy, wary and had mixed feelings about being on an inpatients' ward. Ours was unlocked, a novelty to me. Most of them could have walked out any time. One had been admitted against his will. He was manic-depressive, his latest episode one of many recurrences. His mania (abnormally elated mood) had almost subsided by the time I was tasked with his care. He was cheerful and talkative, just like the woman I had examined for my exam in Heidelberg. The two of us got along like a house on fire, all too well as it turned out. I was instinctively opposed to anything authoritarian and reasoned with him about various dos and don'ts when he requested a weekend pass. He promised to be good and stick to the rules. Naïve as I was, I issued the pass without second thought. Equally without second thought, he bought three brand-new convertibles. His spouse took it in stride, having seen it all before. The car dealer was equally relaxed, and nixed the sale. No harm was done. And I had learned something about "psychotic illness" and how badly it can interfere with judgement.

Most veterans had been admitted for stress-related conditions. They had seen comrades die. Some had walked "point" in the jungle in conditions of poor visibility and a multitude of perils. "Toe popper" mines could explode on a narrow trail at any time. Enemies might attack from the front or rear, from behind bushes and out of camouflaged tunnels. In villages foes looked like friends and friends like foes. One warning sign of an ambush was the metallic click from an AK47 being cocked. Then it was shoot first or hit the deck. Ignoring a click could mean coming second in a firefight. One veteran couldn't stop himself from reacting to clicks as if they were for real, no matter how hard he tried. His comrades kept teasing him, which didn't help his mood. His hypervigilance made perfect sense under Vietnam conditions. It made no sense at all back home, not for him and not to his family. Other anxious vets also couldn't unwind. They slept poorly, had nightmares and became very touchy. Alcohol and drugs had brought them solace first and problems later. Some kept entirely to themselves. During one outing near St. Augustine, they sat silently with a 100-mile stare. They were the most troubled ones, unable to enjoy the balmy breeze and waves breaking in a sandy beach. Detachment had been their main defense in Viet Nam. Now it was destroying their civilian lives. Other vets coped by playing extra hard. I volunteered to play football (rugger) with some brawny marines and learned this the hard way.

An even more disturbing aspect of warfare became clear to me only decades later when a veteran produced a collection of clandestine photos taken after a firefight. They showed half-naked enemy corpses in degrading positions, intended to shock the enemy. The enemy wasn't any kinder to US soldiers. Psychological warfare is nothing new. Mongol warriors placed severed heads on stakes to scare the enemy. *Stuka* bombers screamed down from the heavens during WWII, intent on terrifying troops and civilians below. "Shock and awe" demoralized the enemy at the beginning of the Iraq War. Later on, IEDs and road-side bombs returned the favor. The message is always the same, no matter whose side you are on: You can run, but you can't hide. Stoicism and emotional detachment can be a shield on the battlefield. Back home, it no longer helps. It impedes re-engagement with family and friends who in turn become alienated, feel put off, even rejected by a veteran who seems distant for no apparent reason. The veteran in turn feels abandoned. Nobody understands what he went through and why he doesn't want to talk about distressing memories. Worse than that, he may feel betrayed: Public hostility to the Vietnam War targeted returning GIs during the Sixties and Seventies, men who had risked their very lives for their country. Many had no choice in the matter, except by desertion.

I tried to reason and lent a sympathetic ear. My patients were polite, replied with "yes, sir - no, sir" as if I were an officer, and stayed formal. I couldn't connect with them. Was there an alternative to mere listening that might help? There were several theories to choose from, *organic psychiatry, psychobiology, psychoanalysis and behaviorism.* None was up to the task. Organic psychiatry lacked the technology to diagnose the "minimal" brain injuries soldiers may suffer under bombardment. Medications had unpleasant side effects, and *Prozac* wouldn't' be available for more than a decade. Behavior therapy was in its infancy. Psychoanalysis wasn't offering active intervention. And Adolph Meyer's psychobiology offered little more than chicken soup for the soul. As a wag said at the time: "The two Adolfs are to blame for the lamentable state of American psychiatry; Adolph Meyer by explaining everything as stress reaction and Adolf Hitler by chasing psychoanalysts and their couches across the Atlantic." Treating distressed veterans felt like fighting a dragon with a toothpick. I had less at my disposal than soldiers did during in WWII and Vietnam. German troops used the methamphetamine *Pervetin* to combat fear and fatigue. British pilots used stimulants during the Battle of Britain. And US soldiers spaced out on cannabis, got revved up on "speed" and drowned their sorrows in alcohol. I had nothing better to prescribe. Could a novel version of psychotherapy work? I was more than ready to experiment.

Gainesville's program offered training in a variety of psychotherapies. These included psychoanalysis, *Rogerian* psychotherapy, behaviorism and *Gestalt* therapy. Psychoanalysis was a tool of self-exploration and not a tool of change, suitable only to a clientele prepared to spend years in analysis, not veterans and inpatients in crisis. Carl Rogers believed in "unconditional positive regard" as a way to ease troubled minds. An animal experiment supported this at a long stretch: It introduced "depressed" young monkeys to older experienced "monkey psychiatrists" who then clung to the youngsters until they got better (Scientific American). I couldn't see doing this with burly veterans. Wilhelm Reich's *"Orgon therapy"* was even more far-fetched. Like Freudian psychoanalysis, it blamed anxiety on repressed sexual impulses that were released by allowing forbidden thoughts to enter one's mind. According to Reich, excessive muscle tone also had to be broken to accomplish this. A thorough release would improve orgasms, a proposition I wasn't going to miss. Wilhelm Reich's son-in-law Ollendorf was visiting from Berlin. He'd know more about this than any living person, and his whacky humor appealed to me. During our one and only therapy session, Olly "broke" my muscles for an hour or so by stretching shoulders and hip joints to their physiological limit. I got away sore but unconvinced and turned down his offer to sit in an "Orgon box" for more "release."

Fortunately, more was on offer in the way of psychotherapy training. Two options stood out: *Behaviorism* analyzed problems by observing what people do, where and when they do it and what happens as a consequence. *Gestalt therapy* did something similar by exploring feelings and perceptions "in the here and now," with training made available through active participation in a therapeutic group. Why not try both? - I started with **Ge-**

stalt.

Vincent O'Connell was a PhD psychologist who ran *Gestalt groups* for psychiatric residents. We met weekly for an hour-and-a-half on a strictly voluntary basis, sat in a circle and the brave ones "let it all hang out." Whatever happened in the group stayed in the group, just like Vegas. "*Gestalt*" means "figure" or "shape." *Gestalt* therapy aims to reveal the emotional *Gestalt* of a participant, warts and all, to relieve neuroticism (read emotional kinks). We had to be unreservedly ourselves, hold nothing back and refrain from blaming anyone else for the way we felt and acted. Our perceptions and feelings were our sole responsibility, as were the actions we took. If spending time with someone "made us feel awful," that was our responsibility, not the fault of the companion we had chosen. We weren't victims. We were free agents. By choosing bad company, we chose to feel awful. To get unvarnished feedback about ourselves, we could sit in the "hot chair" that was in the center of the group. I had been brought up to "never let on" and hesitated, then took the plunge. Playing it safe would have felt like cowardice. I talked about homesickness and mixed feelings about "having to" train in Florida, implying that I was a victim of circumstance. Feedback put me straight: "Hadn't I chosen to leave home? Wasn't I free to go back? Choices can be tough, but that's life." I had a good cry and felt strangely elated afterwards, more determined and a little less alone. I was clearer in my head about the implications of my choice between Europe and North America and more determined to make it work. Additional sessions improved my comfort with scrutiny and receiving feedback unfiltered by social convention. Watching others squirm in the hot seat gave me a better feel for discomfiture and evasion and made me a better interviewer. **Roleplay with role reversal** offered greater understanding for the feelings of others. For this we chose a partner "to work with" and revealed to him a concern like a critical comment he had made. After "the offended one" disclosed how he felt, he exchanged seats with the "offender" and roleplayed him.

The "offender" roleplayed the "victim." Role reversal revealed how one perceived the other. Repeated role reversals revised perceptions until both felt fully understood. It was the best empathy training I have ever come across. It's also a useful tool for conflict resolution. - Just imagine Republicans doing this with Democrats, socialists with conservatives and Greens with climate change deniers. It would be quite a party game.

It can also be stressful to the point of requiring a health warning.

By the Sixties, North American society had become highly mobile. Moving from job to job and from town to town broke up relationships that might have grown into friendships under more permanent conditions. Lay groups sprung up in response. They promised to relieve loneliness and alienation by accelerating the slow process of getting acquainted through intense encounters. Stetson College invited John Renick, Rock Cheshire and myself to run such groups on their campus. Many students attended. A few needed "saving" from group pressure and follow-up with therapy. The psychological literature reported emotional breakdowns. To investigate the effects of the groups, we designed a research study with Gainesville students. Molly Harrower, poet and senior faculty member offered outcome assessments through the Rorschach test, a projective method with inkblots, for a pre- and post-group assessment. (She had developed a quantifiable version of this test for the US Air Force years ago.) Her results suggested "positive changes" and a protective effect from the presence of trained therapists, good enough for a brief publication, but not good enough to determine what had caused this change. - For that, a control group with a fake therapy (*placebo*) would have been needed for comparison.

After completing six months' training at the Veterans Administration, I moved to a psychiatric ward at Shands Teaching Hospital. The ward housed people from all walks of life, including a nervous cop who refused to hand over his guns, students hooked on recreational drugs, distressed victims of incest and depressed housewives. A woman with debilitating headaches spent most of her time in bed. Traditional psychotherapy, support from fellow patients, good food, music and art therapy failed to alleviate her "maladaptive response to stress at home." *Gestalt therapy* was a non-starter. "She already had a headache." I wanted better answers to pain and moved to a neurology ward. There I learned how to conduct a proper neurological examination, how to perform a spinal tap, how to assess dementia, paralysis and neural pain. All-night EEG (electroencephalography) research revealed new insights into sleep cycles and their disturbances. - Chronic headache remained a puzzle.

Back on psychiatry at Shands', I finally managed a small but important break-through with another puzzling complaint. A young woman refused to leave home unless her parents accompanied her. Our "working diagnosis" was schizophrenia supposedly caused by Bateson's (now obsolete) "double bind." According to his theory, "schizogenic" mothers invite closeness by saying "yes" verbally and saying "no" non-verbally, thereby stressing the child to the point of psychosis. I scrutinized the interactions between mother and daughter and found nothing of the kind. Fortunately, the behaviorist George Barnard offered a more practical approach. He sidestepped any theorizing and simply asked "what's wrong." That was clear enough: She wouldn't go outside alone. "Then go outside with her and see what happens." I ignored dire warnings from senior staff about the potential dangers of a direct approach and did exactly that. We went for a walk. My patient did just fine. She became neither psychotic, nor did she "act out" (behave crazily) as senior staff had warned. She merely stayed close to me. We went out for more walks and gradually increased our range. Her mobility improved; I don't recall to what extent. - She was probably agoraphobic. And *agoraphobia* may improve with exposure therapy.

Taking my patient for a walk had been the equivalent of a detective's visit to the crime scene. Its psychiatric equivalent, **behavioral assessment** became my guiding light. *Observe, describe and connect the dots, no more and no less.* In Western movies, gun fighters' hands tell you if they'll shoot or not. Words are mere ornaments there. Observe, add nothing and explain away nothing, then connect the dots. To recap: Our young lady wouldn't go out alone. Accompanying her outdoors proved that she was capable of it. Once outdoors, she avoided moving far from her support. What might happen when she tried? What presented the greatest challenge to her? - Nowadays I would ask these questions to confirm (or rule out) a diagnosis of agoraphobia, an anxiety disorder.

The story includes a history lesson. The psychiatrist Westphal described agoraphobia almost a century before my residency. His description was largely forgotten until research into anxiety disorders got off the ground in the Eighties and Nineties. Behavioral assessment had also been around for decades. George Barnard had learned the technique from Joseph Wolpe, a South-African trailblazer. He taught me and I taught others. Fifty years later, behavioral medicine is generally accepted. – Sometimes change flows slowly like molasses.

3.POT, BOOZE AND SNOWBIRDS

"**D**on't Bogart the joint my friend, pass it over to me" went a Sixties song. "Smoke up, expand your mind and grow," counseled a wild-haired Timothy Leary, sitting cross-legged under a palm tree amidst an admiring circle, patron saint to a movement demanding love, peace and liberation. Cannabis smoke mingled with the scent of campfires at a music festival in Crystal Springs. Cannabis smoke hung thickly over an outdoor rock concert with Janis Joplin, frustrating cops searching for the offenders. Respectable citizens entered dreamland with its help, ignoring the ever-present threat of criminal charges. Pot was more than a drug. It was a symbol of rebellion. You hadn't lived if you hadn't held a joint. And if you had, you were an outlaw. Society was trying to sort itself out over it. Five decades later, it's still not done.

To residents on emergency call one thing was perfectly clear. Cannabis kept us busier than we wanted to be. Freak-outs were common amongst novice users. They rushed to the emergency room, terrified and hoping to be "talked down." That took more time than we had. A solid dose of Valium (Diazepam) was more efficient. It stopped a bad trip like a brick wall. Over time, most users became more sophisticated, and the number of drug emergencies dwindled. Perhaps a few users also realized that fooling with one's neurotransmitters can be risky. - Bad trips can lead to panic anxiety and the emergence of psychotic symptoms.

Much has happened since then. The decriminalization of cannabis is following the same pattern as the lifting of Prohibition in 1932. As a first step, medical use was decriminalized. Then prescribing practices loosened, and alcohol became available on an "as needed" basis. Eventually, government discovered the benefits of taxation and made alcohol available for recreational purposes. Cannabis is repeating these same steps, country-by-country and State-by-State. Its legalization is catching up fast with alcohol. Psychedelics may not be far behind.

Alcoholism is a major health problem. It increases the risk of dementia, of heart attacks, strokes, cancer and liver disease. And it comes in many shapes and forms. In Fifties Germany, all our acquaintances drank. Wine tastings were a cherished tradition and the domain of connoisseurs. Alcoholism was jokingly defined as "drinking more than your doctor." When someone went overboard, it was a laugh. Down-and-out alcoholism was unknown in the Germany I grew up in. Liver disease was its best-known manifestation, pancreatitis after exposure to cheap red wine a research subject at the Institute of Pathology. Some of the differences between wine tasters and guzzlers may be sociocultural. Some reflect a biological component. At the Veteran's Administration, Kurt Freund's laboratory had an *"animal model"* for alcohol addiction that suggested the latter. His drunken mice were "just like your old friends." Their behavior fell into three groups. One group took a sip from the nozzle and declined drink after that. The second group liked its booze, but only in moderation. The third stayed glued to the nozzle and went completely blotto.

I hadn't met a human member of the third group before my first encounter in Florida. My patient was bedridden on a medical ward, thin, pale, restless, confused and exuding a fruity smell. His medical workup had been negative and he denied all substance use. I didn't want to insult him by questioning him further and scheduled a second visit with my supervisor. Mike Kehoe was an Irishman wise in the ways of the world and an old hand in such matters. He sniffed the air, then opened the bottom door of the patient's night table without a moment's hesitation. Out tumbled many empty aftershave bottles. The source of the fruity smell was revealed, also the evasiveness that comes with alcoholism. Our patient had the full package. He had the first signs of dementia. He had liver disease and he lacked a social safety net. We patched him up with detoxification, vitamins and a referral to social work. That's all we could do. After this experience I never asked about alcohol use directly. Instead, I'd ask about how many drinks someone "could hold," translating this into an estimate of tolerance. - When someone can "hold a lot" and tolerance is high, alcohol may be one of his major food groups.

I should mention another experience with alcoholism. One patient in a Munich hospital sported a *rhinophyma*, the bulbous red nose that signals chronic use. He wasn't down-and-out like the Floridian man. He looked healthy and had been admitted to hospital for a surgical procedure. He fitted into the second group of Kurt's drunken mice, the moderate but persistent one. His confusion began a day or two after admission. I recognized his withdrawal symptoms, but my management lacked nuance. "Psychiatric symptoms require psychiatric help" was my simplistic rule. I called the men in white coats. They arrived within the hour and carted him off to Haarburg, the mental hospital just outside Munich. The senior doctor chewed me out afterwards: "He would have been just fine with a prescription of red wine." The hospital pharmacy stocked it, and a few glasses would have saved him from upheaval. - The lesson was clear: Treatment should be less disruptive than the illness it's meant to alleviate.

Usually, the arrival of the doctor at the bedside is greeted with a sigh of relief, not so with psychiatric consultants. Only a few welcomed our visit, fearing it might discredit their complaints as **"psychosomatic"** (meaning imaginary). "Psychosomatic" is a fuzzy term I consider outdated. Its history goes back centuries, to the religious belief in an immortal soul. That's a religious construct, not a medical one. When used in a medical context, the term implies an absence of a "physical" problem and the presence of a "psychological" one, a false dichotomy. In reality, all illness affects both body and mind, simultaneously and as one single entity. It's distressing to be ill, to be away from home on a hospital ward and to be uncertain about outcome and cost. The result is as physical as it is mental, and it can delay the recovery. Consequently, psychiatric consultants need to cover more than just mental health. They need to cover physical and socioeconomic health as well, to fully understand a patient's condition. They need to do it tactfully, to dispel any fears a patient may have about symptoms being labeled as "imaginary."

Particular diplomacy was required in the Sixties for a sexual history. You never asked about sex directly, especially not a Southern lady. It was barely proper to ask, "Does your husband still bother you, mam?" With men you could be more direct. Circumspection had gone AWOL however when I interviewed a man of the Cloth. He was in the throes of a new relationship, worried about "failing" and impotent at his first opportunity. To my mind, he needed to feel sexy. And that meant focusing exclusively on the part of his anatomy where he felt this, instead of being distracted by worries about performance. In true *Gestalt* fashion, I went directly to the point. "Be your penis," I advised in a Freudian accent. A puzzled look developed on the minister's face, then an expression of patience and forgiveness. Our therapeutic relationship did not blossom.

Night call presented more challenges. The "Officer of the Day" had to cover all problems at the VA hospital, medical, surgical, neurological and psychiatric, everything that walked through the door. To a novice, this was a terrifying proposition. You had to be a master of all trades, while knowing full well that you were a master of none. Senior doctors were helpful, but unenthusiastic about being woken in the middle of the night. Fortunately, psychiatric emergencies outnumbered all others and nothing life-threatening came my way. A law student filled in as nighttime administrator. His hobby was tracking the "snowbirds" that frequented northern VA hospitals in the summer and migrated south in fall in search for warmer climes. Northern VA administrators alerted him, and he in turn alerted administrators further south to impending arrivals. One night, a "snowbird" wanted a bed, not sometime in the future but " right now." He didn't care for an examination by a Kraut, having seen quite enough of them overseas. When threats didn't produce an instant admission, he got angry. He grabbed me by the throat and the two of us got into a bit of a dance. We pushed and shoved, overturned a table, crashed into a wall and made a lot of noise. Then the cavalry arrived. A senior doctor cleared him medically and the cops arranged his lodging. He spent the night in jail on a hard cot, not in the warm soft bed he had been looking for.

To my relief, night call at Shands was limited to psychiatric emergencies. A novel one was a young lady with **full-blown mania**. She had directed traffic in her birthday suit at a downtown intersection. Cars came to a screeching halt and a traffic jam developed until the cops arrived. They bundled her up and brought her in. Nurses wrapped her in a blanket to prevent another display of charms. I declined her invitation to dance and admitted her against her will, one of the few times I ever had to do this during my entire career. Involuntary admissions required a phone call to the Justice of the Peace. Mine followed a time-honored procedure: "What's up doc?" the Justice asked, sounding a bit sleepy. I described the situation. "That's ok then, doc" he replied and hung up ever so swiftly. - The young lady's case wasn't in the least bit funny. It was dangerous. People with full-blown mania can exhaust themselves completely, collapse and die. Involuntary admission was the only way to save her.

In Gainesville, doctors in training weren't just there to learn.

They were also expected to teach. I dreaded public speaking and avoided it like the plague, unless embarrassed into it. Someone managed to do just that by making soothing noises about "a few student nurses an informal setting," needing to be enlightened on the benefits of psychiatric care. I shouldn't have been so trusting. Instead of a small circle, I found myself on a brightly lit stage in a large hall, filled with chatty young things. Old Glory stood by my side and made the whole thing look frightfully official. I sweated buckets. My heart was racing and I had difficulty breathing as I held my notes with trembling hands. But I survived, climbed down from the stage on wobbly legs and hurried towards the exit, barely hearing a nursing student tell me I was "cute." The experience had me experiment with medications for anxiety. I was prescribing them. Why not try them myself? Diazepam calmed me, slowed my palpitations and eased the feeling of breathlessness during lectures. It also made me drowsy. Amitriptyline (Elavil), the antidepressant of choice at the time, was worse than useless. It made me feel "spacey." The anti-psychotic Chlorpromazine was too sedating. I felt like a wet blanket. Trifluoperazine (Stelazine) had an emotionally steadying effect, but made swallowing difficult after a few doses.

I have paid close attention to complaints about drug side effects ever since.

4. LEARNING TO FEEL: ESALEN AND THE STUDENT HEALTH SERVICE

The Student Health Service occupied a small two-story building smack in the middle of campus. Students could access psychotherapy there free of charge. Two senior staff provided supervision. Our clients were vocal, well informed and a joy to talk to. I could be as busy or un-busy as I wanted to be, played tennis during lunch breaks in the midday sun and frequented the well-stocked university bookstore located just around the corner whenever I felt like it. The bookstore was a God-sent. It offered a smorgasbord of psychology, sociology and psychiatry texts that covered a wide variety of philosophies and orientations. The cat had fallen into the cream. Below is a summary of the **psychotherapeutic tools** I found there, telegram style.

Colby's psychoanalytically oriented psychotherapy (1) has the interviewer home in on the most significant aspect of a client's statements during an interview, then asks follow-up questions accordingly. Question follows question along this path. Unless the client chooses to digress, it will lead to the heart of the matter, be it conflict, fear, loss or love affair. The interviewer maintains absolute neutrality as he listens, keeping his own interests and convictions completely to himself. Nothing must "contaminate" the client's path to self-discovery. Colby's technique worked well in my hands with thoughtful students who wanted to find their own way, but not with students who needed active support. There, Carl Roger's supportive therapy of "I love you, no matter what" was a better fit. Glassner's reality therapy (2) represented a near-opposite to Roger's "unconditional positive regard." It emphasized personal responsibility, problem-solving and the need to face hard facts a client would rather ignore.

Colby's, Roger's, Glassner's and the following psychotherapies differ not only in regards to technique. They also differ in regards to their views on societal versus individual responsibility. *Erich Fromm's* "Sane Society" (3) has a socialist bend. Social problems make people ill, and not the other way around. His non-competitive "sane society" claims to be better for mental health than Glassner's harsh reality where people must fend for themselves. Karen Horney (4) viewed society in feminist ways. She saw womens' lives as inherently conflicted. Society wanted them to be simultaneously both competitive and likeable at one and the same time. Southern ladies in particular had to be "really, really nice" and keep everyone happy through gritted teeth. Horney's analysis of social roles meshed well with *Eric Berne's* transactional analysis (5), a technique that examines conversations in reference to interpersonal hierarchies. Berne's hierarchies come in three basic versions: People can interact respectfully, at eye-to-eye level as "adult to adult". They can interact like a belittling parent would with an ignorant child. And they can interact appeasingly like a submissive child would with a strict parent. Realigning an unequal interaction through therapy can then "de-tox" it. Assertiveness training takes Berne's concept one step further and into the realm of behavior therapy. It uses role-play and rehearsal to help shy people say exactly what they need to say, as adult to adult and without put-downs. It's the individual's responsibility once again to get it right, reminiscent of _Gestalt_ therapy (6), my main interest at the time.

Fritz Perls had founded Esalen, an institute at California's Pacific Coast that offered courses in _Gestalt_ and "personal growth experiences." The courses promised something I could put into practice readily. My friend and fellow resident John Renick felt the same way. We applied, were accepted promptly and the University funded us with jaw-dropping generosity.

Fritz Perls died just before we got to Esalen, but his courses continued. We departed full of anticipation.

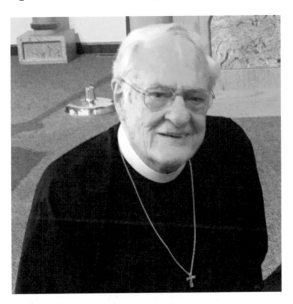

John Renick MD in his most recent incarnation

San Francisco lived up to expectation. It had mountain ranges all around, misty ocean breezes, grand views across Golden Gate Bay, colorful neighborhoods and lots of way-cool people in bell-bottom jeans. We hadn't been there for a day before a stranger invited us to a party. Everyone seemed to spend their time hanging out and hanging loose, chasing new experiences without a care. Rich California wines, the sweet sounds of Santana's "Black Magic Woman" and Mungo Jerry's dreamy "Summertime" got us into the groove. After recovering from the latest party, we rented a large sedan and hit the road a la Jack Kerouac, heading south on California's incomparable Highway One along the Pacific coast. We tasted herb-infused "ambrosia burgers" and luxurious "paradise salads," slept rough in the car, John up front and me stretched out on the back. We idled on sunny hillsides looking out over the Pacific and descended on serpentine roads to sandy beaches. At the gate of Esalen, the sight of a breast-feeding woman greeted us, promising closeness to nature. The Institute's wooden bungalows and meeting rooms sat amongst tall pine trees, perilously close to the edge of steep cliffs. Wisps of cool mist blew up from the sea and large waves crashed into the shore below. Seals and sea lions were hanging out down there. We were hanging out above, feeling as one with nature. Hot tubs provided co-ed conviviality behind a thin curtain of steam. Cold showers calmed those in need. Group sessions had us talking to long-departed parents and relieved us of childhood neuroses. A course on nude massage had us standing in a circle around a female volunteer lying motionless on a slab of old stone, eyes shut. All of us were in our birthday best. I was determined to suppress an unprofessional display of male libido. Pinching myself helped, and recollections of dead bodies on autopsy slabs. I suspect the other males felt the same. A supposedly liberating experience was turning into an exercise of sexual repression. A visit to the cafeteria afterwards reaffirmed societal boundaries: We paid for our meal, as always. – Esalen was mind-expanding and sobering at one and the same time.

John and I flew back to Florida after two weeks of encounter groups, feeling extremely laid back. My new self got rid of his tie, the main sartorial feature that had identified me as a doctor. I was a "transparent self" now, ready for authenticity and self-disclosure. Off-white bell-bottom jeans, sandals and a loose T-shirt were my new uniform. Nobody seemed to mind this except for my British supervisor Mike. He considered it highly "improper."

At the Health Service, students had other worries. They faced the hard reality of the draft and having to go to Vietnam. Homosexuality was still a psychiatric diagnosis then and unacceptable to the military. Some students hoped for an exemption by being diagnosed as "gay." I sympathized, but not to the point of fabricating diagnoses. I called a congressman in Washington on behalf of a particularly distraught student. He lent a sympathetic ear, but had no further comment.

Sometime later the American Psychiatric Association removed homosexuality from its list of Mental Disorders (DSM), and with it this particular escape hatch from the draft.

Change was in the air in many ways in the early Seventies. Signs marking "colored entrances" were fading over rural facilities. Our first black medical student entered Shands Teaching Hospital under police protection. I was too busy being "American" to pay any attention to political strife and the fact that I hadn't met any blacks, apart from the congregation of a small Baptist church. I had read books like "Black Rage" about racial and gender inequality and political dissent, but didn't live any of it. I was too busy fitting in. Then my bubble burst. I had to part from two close friends. John moved to California and my teacher Vincent to Toronto. My favorite cinema closed and I lost access to European cinema. My residency training drew to a close and I felt foot-loose once again, uncertain about next steps. I wasn't ready yet to open a practice and settle down. I also felt homesick. Old Europe with its Gothic cathedrals, baroque chateaux and the feeling of permanence that medieval towns convey was still in my bones. Toronto had felt more "European" than Florida when I visited Vincent there, so why not try it for a year, even if this meant leaving paradise? After all, I could always come back.

Vivian Rakoff at The Clarke Institute (unspeakably re-named *CAMH* years later) interviewed me when I applied. I turned up in California mode, in a T-shirt, bell-bottom jeans and one day late, but precisely at the appointed hour. Maybe the recommendations from Gainesville helped. Maybe Toronto was short of applicants. Vivian grumbled, but he accepted me, and I enrolled for a fourth year of residency training in Toronto. Leaving Gainesville was hard. I was leaving a great university with excellent career prospects. I was leaving those long, lonely roads to the Gulf and the Atlantic, pastures with white, long -horned cattle grazing under giant oaks, the Island Hotel of Cedar Key with its ante-bellum looks where Bessie, innkeeper, retired sociologist and mayor of town mixed her Island Sour whiskeys and fried her crab cakes. I was leaving teachers, friends and a wonderfully laid-back way of life. But off I went, feeling homesick for Florida almost as soon as I arrived in Toronto. I was sorely tempted to move back to Florida after passing my American specialty exams a year later. And I did return many times, but only as a tourist. Florida was changing and so was I. - As an old Chinese man once said so wisely: "You can't descend into the same river twice."

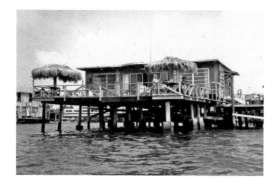

Old Cedar Key

5. A VERY DIFFERENT SCENE: TORONTO, ONTARIO

Montreal had been my first choice amongst Canadian universities. It had the Allan Memorial Institute, cafés, bistros, wine bars, lots of history and old-world charm. But La Belle Province required another rotating internship and a Medical Board exam. Both had to be in French, and I was far from fluent. I considered work a Germany university. I was licensed there, but my American psychiatric training wasn't recognized. I also wasn't in the mood for the serfdom of another residency in Germany. Ontario had the best offer. It recognized my training, and one more year of residency there would qualify me for its Medical Boards and for the Canadian specialty exams. Only the frigid Canadian climate caused some doubt.

To keep my options open, I applied for a renewal of my US visa. I was an odd duck, a German national who had thrown away a US immigration visa and moved to the Great White North. The consul was flabbergasted by my choice. "What' ya doin' up here?" he asked loudly enough for everyone to hear, then issued a visa for unlimited re-entries. Thus reassured, I settled down for a year of Canadian residency. Toronto had museums, an opera house, concert halls, art cinemas, expat communities from all over the world, ethnic food markets and an internationally recognized university. The blue expanse of Georgian Bay and the rugged beauty of the Canadian Shield were just hours' away. It lacked a coffee culture though, and the State-run wine shops had you select your purchases from a printed list without any detailed labelling, an absolute no-no to an oenophile. I also wasn't allowed to import my own wine, as I had in Florida. Thankfully, lots of coffee houses dot today's neighborhoods, and we even have something called the Rare Wine Store.

The powers that be assigned me to St. Michael's Hospital in downtown Toronto. St. Mike's had a timeworn charm with its neo-gothic architecture, nuns in starched habits and a cafeteria that smelled like a granny flat. Its Friday special, Shepard's pie, invited impudent questions about who killed the shepherd. Nearby was the Eaton Center, a very urbane mall with a domed glass ceiling that became invaluable for the exposure therapy of agoraphobics. A Greek hole-in-the-wall restaurant had diners selecting lunches from pots bubbling on the kitchen stove. An Italian dining hall sported waiters in Roman togas. The Underground Railroad offered Southern-style barbecued ribs, black-eyed peas, okra and a "mess" of greens, a good spot for Southern nostalgia. And a German *Gasthaus* combined faux Tudor looks with dark beer and plates piled high with kraut, ham hocks, schnitzels and sausages. I felt almost at home.

The department at "St. Mikes" was less eclectic than the department in Gainesville, but tolerably so. Psychoanalytically-oriented psychotherapy was king. Other psychotherapies were tolerated but not taught. Behavior therapy was thought to be "untried." *Gestalt* smacked of counterculture and raised eyebrows. Residents practiced diagnostic "formulations" to explain the intra-psychic mess of unconscious desires and conflicts that we supposedly harbor. We studied the Diagnostic Manual of the American Psychiatric Association (DSM) and followed its criteria to the letter, much in contrast to my training in Florida. My early efforts attracted little critical acclaim. I failed to see the point of classifying anything beyond the treatment it required. Psychotics got antipsychotics and support. Neurotics got anxiolytics, antidepressants and psychotherapy. Period. Diagnostic classification beyond the basics seemed superfluous, unless it was for clinical research. - There detailed classification is indispensable, or all sub-types of a disorder would end up in the same pot. And that would hinder the development of more specialized therapies.

A second unofficial classification was based on social criteria. The more affluent and more educated were candidates for psychoanalytically-oriented psychotherapy and saw mostly senior staff. The poor, the ones with somatic (bodily) complaints and psychotic disorders saw residents, an allocation that failed to reflect their need for experienced clinicians. There was plenty of supervision though and room for innovation. John Salvendy started a walk-in clinic modelled after Arnold P. Goldstein's "Psychotherapy for The Poor" (7). The "Wednesday Clinic" was located in a disused chapel, which gave it a devotional feel. To trainees, it offered clinical experience with "rubbies" (people drinking rubbing alcohol) and street people with chronic psychoses. To its clients, it offered psychiatric, occupational and social services without requiring a formal commitment. A valid Ontario health card guaranteed access. A social worker would help with the paperwork if someone didn't have one. Nervous newcomers could sit quietly in a corner by themselves, have a cup of coffee and leave again. They could talk to a doctor, nurse or social worker and get a referral to specialist, benefits that would have been difficult to access by any other means. Some clients formed lasting attachments. One alcoholic woman continued to see me until she died of pancreatic cancer.

The limited scope of our care stood in stark contrast to the treatments the "real doctors" could offer in medicine and surgery. They had lab tests and x-rays to diagnose an illness, operations and antibiotics to get rid of it. We had nothing of the kind. Thankfully some cracks showed through the "real doctors'" seeming omnipotence. Diabetics wouldn't follow their pre-scribed diet. Post-operative patients would get "claustrophobic'" in their hospital bed. Cardiac patients would avoid rehabilitative exercise for fear heart attacks. Some refused to leave the safety of the ICU for the same reason. Others reacted in opposite ways, insisting that nothing was wrong with them (a phenomenon called "denial"). They left the ICU against medical advice. Inex-plicable paralyses, numbness, confusion and pains baffled even the most experienced neurologists. A psychiatric consultation could be useful in many of these cases. It could identify psychi-atric disorders, sort out fears, misconceptions and plain old lack of communication.

My first assignment at St. Mike's was on the consultation service, the place where psychiatry and medicine meet and sometimes clash. Donna Stuart, then chief resident, later Chair of Women's' Health and recipient of the Order of Canada, showed me the ropes. She refined my diplomatic skills in a territory where psychiatric consultants know less medicine than the physicians who seek their assistance.

My first challenge was gaining patients' trust. I was there for an honest second look. "Four eyes see more than two" was the man-tra. Consulting was "a detective's job" that looks at a diagnostic puzzle through a different lens. Why did a headache, a bowel symptom or palpitations occur only in one setting, but not in others? Why was a drug "not working?" Was it not taken as prescribed? Did it cause side effects the patient did not dare com-plain about? Has someone looked at the whole patients, not just at one particular illness? A revolving door scenario can easily develop unless someone ties up all those loose ends. The alterna-tive is a chain of referrals from one specialist to another, without "the buck" stopping anywhere, a frustrating process that An-drew Malleson described in "The Medical Runaround" (8).

Sometimes a simple solution hides in plain sight.

The hospital environment was the culprit on this occasion. A boy had suffered severe burns on a large part of his body. After a week's confinement to intensive care, he developed inexplicable confusion and restlessness. I sat down besides the heavily bandaged lad, gave my name and explained what I was trying to do. He was wide-eyed and terrified, didn't know where he was, what time it was, why he was there or where his parents were. Instinctively I re-oriented him. I explained what the nurses and doctors were doing and why. He calmed down after half an hour of this and talked more coherently. I felt like Moses on the mountain. He was suffering from sensory deprivation and sleep loss. The ICU was too noisy for restful sleep. It lacked any indicators of day or night. A multitude of monitors were beeping. Staff was rushing back and forth amongst patients in various stages of agony. Subsequently staff provided the lad with a watch and took care to maintain his orientation. - Modern ICUs are much better at keeping people oriented. They provide a quieter environment, natural light with a normal day/night cycle and semiprivate beds whenever possible.

Night call is the bane of every big-city resident. We endured it on a rotating basis, sleeping fitfully in a Spartan duty room until a phone call jolted us awake. I could watch myself getting conditioned Pavlovian style by the ring of the telephone's bell. After a few jolts, I could only doze until dawn greeted my bleary eyes. Even angels get testy when sleep-deprived. One night a novice operator patched through a call that wasn't even remotely part of night-call duties. "I can't sleep," declared a tremulous voice. "Now I can't sleep either" was my grumpy reply. I was hopping mad at the operator who had connected the call, got out of bed and wandered downstairs to the emergency room, seeking solace in shared misery.

St. Mikes is in a part of town that harbors social problems galore. Threats of self-harm and suicide were common. Drunks abused staff, but couldn't be turned away until a thorough examination established that a discharge was medically safe. Psychiatric residents had to interview people who didn't want to talk to them, to rule out risk of suicide and a danger to others. They had to distinguish the merely irritable from the potentially violent, the merely suspicious from the paranoid, diagnose various kinds of cognitive impairment from alcoholism, dementia and psychosis, then make arrangements for follow-up. They had to parse admissions to their crowded inpatient unit and bargain with residents-on-call at other hospitals for a bed, when their own were full (to my mind the responsibility of hospital administrators). And on the following morning their exhausted self would return to "normal duties," a case study in sleep deprivation.

My second rotation of the year was on inpatients. Like Gainesville's, St. Mike's inpatients' was unlocked and offered a "therapeutic environment" with medication, supportive group psychotherapy, occupational rehabilitation, and social services. It wasn't the Ritz, but it offered refuge to people in crisis. A mere change in tapestry didn't solve their problems though. Crises on the ward had to be defused and everybody had to be kept happy with their stay until they were well enough to leave, this with people who are unhappy by definition. As one of my colleagues quipped: "The ones in hospital want to get out, and the ones outside want to get in." Most did stay the course, with one notable exception. One afternoon the police brought in a man with a bad leg for observation. He was a sturdy fellow, seemingly confused and barely able to walk. And then, when no one was looking, he got better suddenly, ran down the stairwell, out onto the street and into a waiting get-away car. A police detective arrived on the double and the bitter truth emerged. Our escapee was an Oscar-deserving malingerer with an impressive criminal record. It fell to me to explain that neither had we been informed of the criminal aspects of the case, nor could we unmask a skilled malingerer in a matter of hours. And an unlocked psychiatric ward can't hold a hardened criminal.

The snows of my first Canadian winter lasted well into April. What had I done to myself, moving to this frost-bitten neighborhood and a bargain-basement salary? But I hung in there, studied and studied, bulky textbooks supported by an affectionate cat purring on my lap. And I made it. By the end of summer, I had survived six years of medical school, two years of internship, four years of psychiatric residency, the Royal College specialty exam and the LMCC general medical exam. I was qualified now for independent psychiatric practice and ready to be let loose on all of Ontario. Qualification didn't solve one nagging problem though, summed up by a rude German pun: "Surgeons know nothing, but they do a lot. Neurologists know a lot, but they do nothing. And psychiatrists know nothing and do nothing." - It would take me the better part of a professional lifetime to find an answer to it.

6.ON STAFF AT LAST

P assing the medical and the psychiatry boards added two feathers to my cap. Passing the American boards in New York added a third. The University of Toronto added a fourth by appointing me lecturer with a full-time staff position. Now that I had the headgear, how would I survive? Would I publish or perish? Would I make a decent living? For the latter, I had to produce "billable hours" just like a lawyer would. If I spent more hours on billable services, I would make more money. If I spent more hours on teaching and research, I would make less, potentially a lot less. Should it be like Berthold Brecht's "Erst kommt das Fressen, dann die Moral" (Grub first, morals later), or like wearing the hair shirt? It wasn't entirely my choice. When the departmental chair asked you to lecture, you couldn't refuse without losing favor. With perfect logic, junior staff gave more lectures and senior staff made more money.

Psychiatry Associates, fondly known as "Psychotic Associates" amongst the lower ranks, ran the business end of the department at St. Mike's. Associates paid the bills and distributed the funds our billable hours had generated, this according to a predetermined formula. All staff psychiatrists could vote in its monthly meetings. "Psychotic Associates" was like the United Nations. Two Aussies, one Hungarian-Austrian, one Yugoslav, one Canuck from Trinidad, two Brits and one German held "frank and open" discussions over lunch, dinner and the coffee machine, sometimes also in a dark corner of the hallway. Most voted in support of the chief's priorities. Occasionally, they rebelled. Once a flurry of sugar bags disrupted the chief's lengthy speech. On another occasion, the chief intended to sequester extra funds from our billable hours, to hire yet another psychoanalyst. This time, a band of dissidents resorted to the subversive use of Robert's Rules of Order. A vote over an ad-hoc bonus payment to all members appeared at the top of next meeting's agenda. It was hugely popular and passed after minimal debate. It also de-funded the chief's pet project, to his exclusive surprise. - Psychotic Associates may have run a distant second to the resourcefulness of parliamentary committees. It still provided a lovely training ground.

Money wasn't the only ticklish issue in the department. Who would treat what kind of client was another. Insight-oriented psychotherapists needed clients that were introspective, educated, vocal and enjoyed flexible hours. Working with them was more profitable and less crisis-prone than working with the poor. It also had a downside. Too many psychotherapists were chasing too few "suitable" clients. The reverse was true for the "unsuitables," impoverished clients with severe anxiety, depression, pain and "psychosomatic" complaints. They had no place to go. Fortunately, several staff psychiatrists redressed this imbalance. Josip Divic introduced a health questionnaire that included physical complaints, thereby widening the focus of intake interviews to physical illness, "psychosomatic" disorders and severe anxiety. Donna Stewart's work at St. Mikes and later as Chair in Women's Health included gender-specific concerns and led to the founding of a women's' clinic in Saudi Arabia. John Salvendy's Wednesday Clinic improved treatment adherence by an impoverished clientele that was too disorganized to keep appointments made weeks in advance. I opened a headache clinic that was booked to the hilt by "psychosomatic" clients who couldn't get help elsewhere. It wasn't a departmental priority though and was closed twice "for lack of space." Finding a confrere in Richard Swinson for my interest in behavior therapy helped me over this setback. Richard was a quietly determined Englishman who arrived in Canada roughly at the same time as myself. He furthered my research interests for decades at three different hospitals, first at St. Mike's, then at Toronto General Hospital (TGH, later part of UHN) and finally at CAMH (originally named the Clarke Institute). At TGH, his administrative skills and an eclectic chief (Alastair Monroe) allowed us to open Canada's first university-based Anxiety Disorders Clinic. (It had existed unofficially before at St. Mikes.) Research on anxiety disorders earned it international recognition. Richard was the anchor that kept me in Toronto and connected me to a critical mass of collaborators that enabled future research on PTSD and pain.

7.FIRST DIPS: INVESTIGATING A HEADACHE

Remember the headache lady from Florida? Her pain was so severe that she retreated to bed in a darkened room. That's common in migraine and severe tension headache. Millions have this problem. The cause of headache was unclear back then and medication of little help. At St. Mike's, some headache patients were eager to try something, anything, to find a way forward. And so was I. But how? There was nothing abnormal to see beyond complaints of pain and a perfectly understandable moodiness. I kept stabbing into the dark until, one lucky day, I bumped into a big surprise. It wasn't what I had been looking for, but never mind. You take what you can get, when you get it.

Two theories of chronic headache seemed worth a closer look. One was a theory about **tension headache.** "The monkey in the rain forest" was its animal model: Monkeys hunch their shoulders in foul weather to keep off rain and wind. We humans supposedly do the same when our emotional "weather" turns foul. If we do it for too long, we get sore. Over time, persistent tension exhausts our muscles, so the theory continues. They become chronically painful.

In **migraine headache**, vascular (blood vessel) constriction is considered the culprit. "Getting cold feet" may be a sign of it. Cold feet suggest unease and a readiness to cut and run. If vasoconstriction can be prevented, so the migraine theory went, then an episode of migraine headache might also be prevented. – Note the many "ifs" and my omission of modern theories about headache.

Theories are useless without supporting evidence. I needed to open a "window" into the physiological mechanism of headache to evaluate the two theories. Police investigators use such a "window" to out a liar. The "lie detector" tracks changes in a suspect's respiration, heart rate and sweating in response to probing questions. The investigator homes in on these bodily signs of distress. Whenever distress increases, she digs deeper, until the suspect is cornered. (Caveat: "Lie detectors" can get "false positives" in nervous subjects and "false negatives" in people who manage to stay calm.)

I restricted my headache investigation to muscle tone and peripheral temperature. A variety of monitors were commercially available for this purpose.

The idea of physiological monitoring in headache was novel, completely untried and unlikely to attract funding for the high-tech versions we see in operating rooms, intensive care and police departments. A poor man's solution was available from a laboratory in Montreal. It sold "biofeedback" equipment, as monitor-aided relaxation techniques were called in the Seventies. The equipment was relatively cheap and good enough for my purposes. It monitored muscle tone and peripheral temperature and fed them back to the volunteer via a visual display and an auditory signal, both in real-time. **Real-time feedback** improves control over functions that would be haphazard without it, just like mirrors improve shaving and applying make-up. Theoretically, biofeedback loops would thus enable volunteers to lower muscle tone and increase peripheral blood flow. And maybe, just maybe, this might relieve their headaches as well.

The St. Mikes hospital research committee agreed to fund the purchase of a temperature and a muscle-tension monitor (EMG) for a pilot study. I added a monitor for sweating (galvanic skin response or GSR) from my personal funds. - I was off to the races.

For temperature feedback I attached the sensor to an index finger and connected it to the monitor. That closed the feedback loop. My volunteer could literally hear her finger cool down or warm up and see it happen on a visual display. I was my first guinea pig and a successful one. I raised my finger's temperature by some seven degrees after hour or two of trying. Most volunteers did equally well. Monitoring muscle tension was just as straightforward. I attached EMG electrodes to the dorsal neck muscles, the temple and forehead while my volunteer relaxed in an easy chair. The pitch of the feedback sound from the monitor increased as muscle tension increased. It decreased as muscle tension dropped, changes confirmed by movements of a needle on the visual display. The volunteers learned to relax nicely, some a bit too well. On occasion a gentle snore emanated from the lab. Clearly, people could be taught to relax with the help of a feedback loop. Now to the million-dollar question: Could my volunteers control their headaches by controlling muscle tone and peripheral temperature?

A majority of my volunteers did indeed report "improvement" with biofeedback. But here's the rub. Chronic headaches wax and wane over time, just like most other chronic ailments. They improve and worsen in an up-and-down pattern that only observation over time can reveal. Unless these spontaneous ups-and-downs are accounted for, it's impossible to tell if biofeedback really helped. Effects from the timing of treatment must also be considered. When biofeedback is offered when a headache is at its worst, improvement is likely, no matter what you do. The headache is merely completing its usual up-and-down cycle. Unsophisticated observers however may misread this as a treatment benefit. How then can we tell the difference between spontaneous variation accented by timing and genuine treatment effects? It's a million-dollar question that needs asking whenever an ailment follows a spontaneous up-and-down pattern. Thousands of happy clients may be thanking their therapist for nothing more than her company, spending money they could spend better on something else.

I didn't worry all that much about timing and spontaneous variation in my trial design. Mine was an "open label pilot," designed for nothing more than a first look. Had it demonstrated major benefits, a larger **placebo-controlled trial** would have been worthwhile as a sequel. That wasn't the case. A controlled trial is only worthwhile when the odds of success are good. It would have to measure average symptom levels over weeks and months before treatment, to establish a "baseline" of headache frequency and severity for later comparison with treatment effects. It would have to include a control group with a fake treatment. It would have to keep both, the treatment group and the control group, in the dark ("blind") in regards to allocation. And it would have to keep assessors equally "blind" to treatment, to guard against their inherent desire to find success. - Controlled trials are cumbersome and expensive, but a necessary evil. An absence of controls leaves too much room for doubt.

Failure is grist for the mill. Learn and move on, with gritted teeth if need be, but move on. *Galvanic skin response (GSR)* monitoring had opened a third window into the physical symptoms of anxiety, my favorite subject. It works the same way as temperature and muscle tone biofeedback and is simpler to use. It became useful by chance when a headache patient tried it during an exploratory interview. I attached a GSR monitor to her index finger that emitted a ticking sound that sped up and got louder whenever her sweating increased. I enquired about neutral subjects first, then about family. The ticking sped up. I homed in some more on family matters, and the ticking grew into a high-pitched scream. I changed back into neutral territory and the scream subsided. I changed back once again to family matters, and the scream returned. Something discomfiting was going on there, something she hadn't disclosed.

The GSR experiment demonstrated to my client that distress has physical consequences, and this reduced her resistance to psychotherapy for somatic symptoms.

And then I got really lucky. I tried GSR with **accident survivors**.

Fast forward to the Eighties. I was riding the subway on my way home when a man nudged me in the ribs, pointing at a woman napping on her seat. She was his spouse, he said, and I had treated her nine years earlier (in the early Seventies) with great success. Feeling keen as always on a success story, I conducted a follow-up interview on the spot, results confirmed later by Jean Martin, our nurse at the Mental Health Clinic and guardian of the coffee maker. Jean had assisted me when I treated the client. She also kept in touch with her subsequently, creating the kind of follow-up most therapists can only dream of. The client's complaint had been head- and neck pain after a car accident. Biofeedback did not help, but it demonstrated the physiological aspects of her anxiety. And that led her to believe that anxiety aggravated her pain. Logically, I suggested then that we get into a car to check this out. This was more easily said than done. She had refused car rides ever since her accident. They terrified her, she said, but she would be prepared to try one under sedation and in the company of her (then) boyfriend. I agreed, and gave her a strong intravenous dose of an anxiolytic before the ride. Jean and I half-carried her to my car under the suspicious eye of a policeman. I put her in the back seat beside her boyfriend and drove her through traffic for some two hours. I also snapped some Polaroid shots as proof that she had done it. She had little recollection on follow-up because of the amnesic effects of the anxiolytic, but the Polaroid shots convinced her that she could do it again. We repeated the procedure several times, reducing her anxiolytic dose each time, until she rode medication-free. Long-term success was nothing short of dramatic. She became able to travel alone and without restriction. She also believed that her pain was better by the end.

This was breaking new ground, as other researchers have confirmed. I replicated the procedure over the following decades with many other survivors of traffic accidents, mostly without sedation. Their fears improved. Pain rarely did. Years later I collated my observations with observations by Richard Swinson and published them as a "first" in the Canadian Journal of Psychiatry. Publication of a treatment manual by the American Psychological Association followed, then a screening test for **accident phobia** (excessive and counter-productive fear of accidents), the Accident Fear Questionnaire (AFQ).

One of my colleagues, Bill McCormick, published a description of **declining dose desensitization** for phobias. Subsequent research has shown that exposure therapy (confrontation with feared situations) may actually be more effective without prior tranquilization than with it. It's been useful in my hands though. It makes it easier for severely phobic people to have a go at a therapy they would refuse otherwise.

One piece of advice to those tempted to try this on a friend: Don't do it without the help of an experienced physician or psychologist. Exposure therapy is demanding. *Its success depends entirely on the willingness of the phobic to confront fear directly, repeatedly and for extended periods of time, without interruption until the urge to leave has abated*; or the phobic will get worse, potentially a lot worse. *Exposure should also never be attempted by surprise and never without prior consent. And it is only as good as the behavioral assessment that preceded it*, as I will show below. In other words, not everything is a nail when you hold a hammer.

Some of my clients remained fearful, no matter how much time we spent on the road. Then it was back to the drawing board, to find answers to the obvious question: Why did they fail to desensitize where others succeeded? More precisely, what exactly did they fear in the first place? One example was an executive who used to commute by chauffeur-driven car. He was a classical back-seat driver who kept shouting at his chauffeur in a manner so distracting, the chauffeur threatened to quit. When I did the driving, he shouted less, but that was it. I had to up the ante by getting him to ride blindfolded, to have him surrender all control over car and driver. Then, and only then did exposure therapy find its proper aim. A published analysis of some sixty cases (for the AFQ) revealed this as a common pattern: Most nervous accident survivors fear riding as passengers far more than driving a car themselves. They want to be in control and distrust everybody else.

Some driving fears have nothing at all to do with accident phobia. A fear of driving across bridges and over exposed hills turned out to be agoraphobic in nature. A fear of taking the wheel was puzzling, until I reversed the usual arrangement and had the client chauffeur me. She then had me on the edge of my seat during a series of near misses. Her fear was entirely realistic and not something I could treat. I referred her to a **course in defensive driving**. It covered safe lane changes, proper separation from other cars, not getting "boxed in" by surrounding vehicles and "skid control" on an oil-covered track. On another puzzling occasion I served as impromptu vehicle inspector. A "floating feeling" made this driver feel "unsafe." He was right. His vehicle had wobbly front wheels and loose steering. It wasn't him that needed fixing. Desensitization would have been worse than useless.

A visit to the "crime scene" for a first-hand look often reveals details the client may have missed. It's a vital step before exposure therapy.

8.HIGH ANXIETY, IN THE SKIES AND ELSEWHERE

F ast forward beyond the year two thousand. Fear of flying had been familiar to me from years of practice. Patients had described it, and its treatment had become routine. But still I wondered what it felt like. What made it so intoler-able that giving up travel felt like the only realistic solution? And then my wishes came true. I got the frights myself while flying home from overseas. "Always look at the bright side" sang the Pythons, and here it was, a chance for a first-hand look at my very own flight phobia. It bugged me though. How could this happen to me, a physician with decades of experience? According to the ancient Greeks, the God Pan is to blame for panic. He spread it amongst lonely shepherds in remote hills, and now he spread it to me. The image of a lonely shepherd didn't fit me though. I wasn't lonely, and flying had been second nature to me. I had to admit to a degree of vulnerability though: I have a nervous predisposition (read biological factor). And I have al-ways been mildly claustrophobic, just never to such breath-tak-ing intensity.

Clinical protocol demanded a proper learning history, to eluci-date how I got from mild claustrophobia to a full-fledged case of the frights.

I got the frights briefly in the Seventies on an unventilated plane. Four of us were in Peru at Santiago airport shortly after Pinochet came to power. The airport was chaotic. Passengers were trying to get a flight to "anywhere, just out of here." After an anxious wait and with a bit of bargaining, we boarded our flight to Lake Titicaca high up in the Andes. The plane was completely empty, and it didn't take off as scheduled. It sat on the tarmac in the boiling sun, with doors closed. No announcement explained the delay, and we couldn't tell if a pilot had come aboard. The air conditioning also wasn't on, and the cabin got stifling hot. I began to feel short of breath and panicky, thought about heat stroke and other unlovely things, but managed to stop myself. I switched to clinical mode and observed my surroundings with detachment. Eventually the plane took off and I relaxed. The rest of the flight was uneventful and I forgot all about it. Years passed without further mishap. Then, one early morning in the Nineties, I got my second episode. I was flying home from San Francisco after celebrating with family the night before. We parted early in the morning, always a difficult moment for me. I rushed to the airport through slow-moving morning traffic, loaded with caffeine and anxious to make it onto the flight. Once there and while the plane was still taxiing, I got anxious again, felt hot and had trouble breathing. This passed after takeoff, and I forgot all about it. Nothing further happened until just before retirement. That's when the frights really struck. I was flying home from London-Heathrow early one morning after goodbye celebrations the night before. Caffeine had helped me through rush-hour traffic. Then, while the plane was still taxiing, I felt the same old sickly fear in the pit of my stomach. It faded when the plane took off, but this time it returned with growing intensity. I couldn't dismiss it. I had the same thoughts that my clients report: "This is intolerable. What if I can't stop this? How much longer can I hang on?" My fear continued to grow. I was like being sucked into a vortex of unspeakable terror. I felt faint, breathless and my heart was going crazy. I went to the wash-room and splashed cold water on my face. That worked, but only briefly. The next wave hit and I felt pulled under once more. Fortunately, training and experience kicked in. It was "physician heal thyself." I was going to use all I knew from treating clients. I was bloody well going to cope.

I countered the closed-in feeling by inhaling and exhaling slowly from the depth of my stomach, as if asleep. A blast of air from the ventilation system helped some more. I gave myself a talking-to: "This is silly. Anxiety doesn't kill" and "counting the minutes and hours until arrival only makes matters worse." I resolved to stay put indefinitely, no matter what, relaxed neck and shoulders and tried to get into a book. This worked for a while, but the frights returned whenever my concentration slackened. And then it dawned on me that focusing on how I felt was a big part of the problem. A reality check was readily available: Nobody else on the plane was freaking out. Everybody looked perfectly relaxed. Some were snoozing. My surroundings were safe. Nothing had reached inside me to cause this existential dread. It was entirely of my own making. I had associated flying with confinement and confinement with asphyxiation. I gave myself another talking-to: I must break this association through repeated reality checks and by treating the frights as something that I generated myself. I must displace fright with fight to subdue this horror, breathe like a relaxed person, stop staring down the rabbit hole and do something interesting instead.

I got through the San Francisco flight all right, then realized that I had acquired the "**fear of fear**" that Claire Weekes (9) describes so well. She had it nailed: Nobody in his right mind would want a repetition of the frights (panic anxiety), but there's no guarantee they won't recur on the next flight. That creates a paradox: Because there's no guarantee, I'd worry. And the more I'd worry and the harder I'd try to prevent the frights, the more attentive I would become to the slightest twinge of fear. And that would drop me right back into the rabbit hole again the moment I felt trapped inside a plane. - My fear of the frights would trigger more frights.

How could I unlearn now what I shouldn't have learned in the first place? A story made the rounds in the early days of behavior therapy. Someone with a bad case of the frights (full-fledged agoraphobia in his case) was feeling hopeless about ever getting better. He felt trapped in a way of life he couldn't accept and decided to put an end to it all by suicide. Instead of the usual means, he chose poetic justice. He went to a lonely hilltop, the scariest place he could think of, expecting to die there from sheer terror. He got there, waited, and nothing happened. Instead of trying his best to avoid the frights, he had challenged them head on. He had invented a technique called "**flooding with paradoxical intent**." He had defeated the fear of fear by saying "I don't care! Bring it on!" Years later a woman called into a CBC radio talk show with the very same idea. She was convinced that dealing with the frights required accepting death, even welcoming it. According to her, only a near-suicidal determination would defeat the frights once and for all.

Who will be this determined, you ask? Flooding with paradoxical intent may be a powerful intervention. It's also a bit harsh. I like my comforts as much the next guy. What else could I try? Was there anything more genteel? The study on panic disorder described in a later chapter offers a hint. Close to one-quarter of our panicky volunteers in the study improved without getting any treatment. What had happened? The study protocol required complete abstinence from **alcohol and caffeine** for two weeks before enrolment. That's when their improvement occurred. Here's my theory (and it's only a theory): Nervous people are on a hair-trigger. Even moderate amounts of caffeine and the mildest form of alcohol withdrawal before departure can aggravate nervousness. Nowadays my flight preparations include a week's abstinence from alcohol, and no caffeine on the morning of departure. I also keep my "emotional temperature" low by observing a leisurely schedule. And I have a dirty secret: I carried

an anxiolytic on board for years. It can terminate the frights, should that be absolutely needed. I never had to take it though. Just carrying it on board sabotaged my "fear of fear." My clients had similar experiences. - I guess I am just like my patients.

I have flown many times since, initially with apprehension, later on with lessening concern. Practice helped. I still carry my pharmacological crutch when I am edgy. A full recovery requires flying without having one in your pocket, while also adding paradoxical intent. I prefer flying with my crutch until I manage to forget it, just like most of my clients did.

Not all flight phobics are created equal. The likes of me have their fear of flying grafted onto **claustrophobia**. Others fear travel far from home. They are **agoraphobic**, and flying takes them too far for comfort from their "safe place." **Disaster phobics** are different again. They get the frights when aircraft wings wiggle in rough weather and engine sounds change. They fear their plane might crash. These distinctions matter greatly. You can try desensitization therapy until blue in the face if you "target" the wrong fear. In the Seventies Air Canada allowed a VIP client and myself onto the flight deck of a parked Boeing 747, to get her back into her old flying routine. Staff was most reassuring, explained the many safety features of the plane and let us stays as long as we wanted. It didn't help one bit. Safety wasn't my client's worry. Being far from home was, as I came to realize. She was agoraphobic and that requires different help.

Here's a golden rule: **Behavior therapy is only as good as the preparatory assessment.**

Anxiety Disorder

comes in many shapes and guises. It affects some eighteen percent of the North American population annually, which makes it the most common psychiatric disorder in the general population. (Some databases list depression as more common.). DSM includes a list of different anxiety disorders, including **generalized anxiety disorder** ("the worry warts"), **illness phobia** (ceaseless worry about all kinds of things), **animal phobia** (fears of snakes, bats, cats, dogs etc.), **social phobia** (fear of negative evaluation), **obsessive-compulsive disorder** (ceaseless counting, checking and collecting), **needle phobia** (faintness from injection) and **agoraphobia** (fear of public places and going far from home). Anyone can get an anxiety disorder. It's part genetic (according to twin studies), part learned behavior. It changes lives and is easily overlooked. Anxious people don't act "crazily" or get more aggressive than the average person. They are anxious about something going wrong, and most hide their condition as best they can. Some get depressed, and some believe they are suffering from an undiagnosed medical condition like heart disease.

Panic disorder (with or without full-fledged agoraphobia) is a particularly severe variant of anxiety disorder. In the USA and Europe, its one-year prevalence (cases observed over one year) is roughly 1.7% of the general population (National Institute of Mental Health). People with panic disorder get the frights unexpectedly (DSM). They are unaware of triggers. People with **agoraphobia** are aware of triggers. They get the frights in places they fear already, like crowds and being too far from the safety of home. Westphal's description from the year of 1871 is identical to the contemporary "panic disorder with agoraphobia" of DSM. His three young men experienced the same sudden terror and the same fear of empty streets and the "*agora*" (Greek for meeting place) that our agoraphobics describe.

Phobias represent survival fears in one way or another that were useful at times like the Stone Age. It was unwise then to go far from home and one's clan, reckless to be all-alone in a strange place where getting back to safety might take too long. You wouldn't let surrounded by a crowd of strangers either, not without the means for a quick escape. Bolting like a frightened horse might have been the best option whenever things looked risqué. That's rarely practical nowadays, but still part of everyone's survival skills. It's just more intense and less controlled in phobic individuals. Phobias can be mild and it can be crippling. Chances are that many readers know someone with it, someone who "needs to leave" suddenly, someone who "doesn't like" small animals, the cinema or crowds. Mild phobia can remain unrecognized for years, until a change at work requires travel to new places, or when a medical disorder like irritable bowel or asthma intensifies the need for safety from mishaps.

The Toronto subway was one of the most feared places for my agoraphobic clientele. My company made it easier for them to go there for **exposure therapy**. I would choose a graded approach, sit next to a client on the subway at first, then several seats away. Then I would ride in the next car and on the next train, until the client could ride unassisted. The Eaton Center in downtown Toronto offered a menu of other situations that agoraphobics fear. It offered crowds, heights, elevators and narrow passageways, perfect for exposure therapy. Group treatment offered economy of time and the added benefit of mutual encouragement. **Independent practice** without the reassuring presence of a therapist or companion is mandatory before eventual "graduation." Without it, the need for support cannot be broken and the client continues to depend on help.

People with **posttraumatic stress disorder** (PTSD) also get the frights, but more in tune with contemporary reality than agoraphobics. They have experienced a modern version of Stone Age danger, be it combat, accident, assault or a terrifying emergency. Their frights are "triggered" by reminders and fears of a repetition, and require care that's different from that for other phobias.

A full **recovery** from the frights requires more than reducing symptoms down to zero. Quality of life must be restored before success can be declared. Someone with agoraphobia should be able to travel without undue distress as far as he may choose. Whatever constitutes that depends on a client's hopes and ambitions. Hope can be a moving target. When someone loses hope and gives up, very little will happen in therapy. When hope and ambition stay alive, a lot can happen. To name one shining example: An agoraphobic man had been unable to travel alone beyond Toronto's downtown core. He wanted to work abroad. And he did. Years after we had parted, a small parcel from Down-Under arrived with his thanks. It contained the impression of a fossilized fish in a stone. It's still on my desk, memento to his dream come true. Only a small percentage of clients accept exposure therapy as full-fledged as this man did. It requires great fighting spirit and never forgetting why one is in the fight. Therapists can support, encourage, nudge and push. Only a sustained vision of a better future provides the pull that helps a client go all the way.

9.SOCIAL ANXIETY: WHAT WILL PEOPLE THINK?

J ust about everybody knows social anxiety. It's baked into our society. Teens feel it when they log onto their social media page. Singles feel it on a first date. Speakers, actors and performers feel it when the curtain rises. It's all about being judged and considered wanting. The flip side of it is ambition and needing to be liked. How can one get over a bad case of it?

Social anxiety stretches across a continuum, from apprehension and worry to full-fledged **social phobia.** The American Psychiatric Association's diagnostic manual (DSM) defines the latter as a **"fear of negative evaluation"**. You fear humiliation, ridicule and rejection and get stage fright whenever you feel on display. At a less extreme and more common level, you are just thoroughly uncomfortable.

My dear old gran exemplified the latter. She grew up in a small German wine-growing community during the early Nineteen-hundreds. Everything is cheek-by-jowl there and acceptance matters greatly. You depend on your neighbor, carpenter, butcher and your grocer. They in turn depend on you. Everybody knows everybody's business and everybody gossips. Angering someone in such circumstances can make life very difficult.

"What will people think" was gran's trademark expression. It summed up her worries and her dilemma. She wanted people to think well of her. She also was unsure because she couldn't tell what they thought. And that's uncomfortable for anyone who wants acceptance.

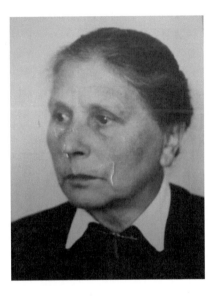

My gran Anna, looking concerned

My gran did her best to make sure. She cleaned, cooked, ironed, prayed for sinners like me and made the best dumplings in town. This guaranteed her standing in the family. Our standing in the community's was harder for her to gauge. All she could do was to fuss. "Murphy's Law," the rule of "whatever can go wrong, will go wrong," could have been her invention. She worried about "the life I was leading," fussed about my manners, my rumpled pants, my haircut and what people will think if I went into town "looking like this." The popular BritCom "Keeping Up Appearances" represents a different version of the same angst. The lead, "Mrs. Bucket," also wants acceptance. But, instead of worrying about what people might think, she ploughs straight ahead. She fakes a posh accent, insists on having her name pronounced "bouquet," and pushes candlelight dinners on important people who would rather be elsewhere. Her under-assertive neighbors don't dare saying "no" to her face. That would be too embarrassing. Instead, they run and duck behind hedges to avoid her overbearing company. The joke is on them as well. Gerhart Hauptmann's describes something similar in his *"Hauptmann von Koepenick."* His colonel is an ordinary man who dons a colonel's uniform. And that's all it takes to order about a town of obsequious bourgeois. In Gottfried Keller's *"Kleider machen Leute"* (clothing makes the man), an impoverished tailor does it again, only more subtly. He cuts himself a fine suit, and that gets him respect from people undiscerning enough to fall for this trick.

Do we know any better? An entire industry dresses us up in the latest fashion. We suffer through slimming diets and undergo plastic surgery to look like movie stars. We buy sleek cars and fancy clothes to look successful. We seek the company of celebrities and seek status by association. Social climbing may be a harmless sport when practiced in moderation. It's a disease when rooted in profound self-doubt. According to Alfred Adler's *"inferiority complex,"* doubting oneself beyond reason leads to "overcompensation," to over-doing in a counter-productive way the normal desire be liked and admired. It's the root cause of over-spending, over-soliciting and being over-sensitive to anything that resembles criticism.

Social phobia is one more step beyond feelings of inferiority. It's far more intense, even paralyzing and like freezing from stage fright. My gran worked hard to please everyone, but she functioned. Mrs. Bucket's ambitions misfired, but she managed to plow on. Someone with an "inferiority complex" may try too hard, brag, con and annoy, but he will keep going. Social phobia is that on steroids. A social phobic is terrified. He freezes in his tracks and can't function. Any deviation from the social conventions of the time can occasion this. The general theme remains consistent: Social phobia an excessive fear about appearing "inadequate" in some shape or form.

The paradox of the *fear of fear* aggravates this in the same way as it aggravates a fear of flying, with one difference. It's not triggered by internal harbingers of emerging panic. It's triggered by feeling at the verge of an embarrassing misstep. A phobic job applicant might tremble slightly during an interview, and he would be hyperalert to it. His *fear of fear* would then kick in, and cause him to tremble a lot more. The same sequence applies to blushing. A blusher's face would turn beet-read as soon as he felt it flush ever so slightly. Most social phobics understand this sequence perfectly well. They just can't stop it. It's as if they were always on stage before a hypercritical audience.

I had one nervous shaker as a client who couldn't bring herself to sign a check in front of a bank teller (this before the days of online banking). The teller might watch her trembling hands with eagle eyes, suspect fraud and call the police. She played it safe and had her friends do her banking for her. Compare her belief to the belief of a friend of mine with Parkinson's disease. She also shakes and doesn't like it one bit. To her though, that's just too bad. No need to hide it. She even teams up with a few others with Parkinson's. They call themselves "the movers and shakers" and raise money for good causes, a striking example for the central role thoughts and beliefs play in social phobia.

The most direct way to defeat social fear is to flaunt your imperfections. A German proverb sums it up: *Und ist der Ruf erst ruiniert, lebt man gänzlich ungeniert.* (Ruin your reputation, and you will be rid of embarrassment.) The therapeutic principle of *"exposure with paradoxical intent"* applies here as well as elsewhere with panic anxiety, if you can handle the discomfort. It's worth it if you can, as in the case of an executive who wouldn't wear his light-colored suit on hot summer days. Sweat stained its fabric visibly whenever he felt on edge, showing him up as the nervous wreck he was. But he was determined. We sprayed his armpits with water until stains showed. He then walked through the clinic's waiting room, to gauge people's reactions. And nobody paid any attention. The same happened later at work, apart from the occasional second look. It was what Frieda Fromm-Reichmann called "a corrective emotional experience," a forceful demonstration of what matters and what doesn't. Cognitive preparation needs to pave the way towards such a direct confrontation with fear: Ask what the consequences would be in a worst-case scenario. Would you get fired? That's unlikely. Would you be the butt of jokes and derision? If so, rehearse this worst-case scenario before your inner eye and practice staring down ridicule and abuse: They don't know any better. They are the fools, not you.

One man had an unusual mix of stage fright and illness fear. He "couldn't swallow" when he felt watched and feared choking as a result. He was about to get married, and that presented him with a situation he couldn't dodge. He would have to sit at the head table, bring a toast to the bride and eat his meal, all this while on full display. His GI specialist convinced him that a little help could solve his problem. Having a meal with him in public right off the bat would have triggered unmanageable anxiety. We met for small lunches at my office instead. We started with yoghurt, moved up the scale to salads, hamburgers and finally tackled stringy beef. My presence helped. He knew I wouldn't let him choke to death. After he was comfortable with this, he struck out on his own, practiced at restaurants, first alone and then in company. And that got him through his wedding.

Therapy can go wrong for many reasons. Overconfidence is one. Buoyed by my success with the groom who couldn't swallow, I arranged to meet with a group of women who also feared eating in public. I had done it once. I could do it again, or so I thought. We would meet at a small restaurant in a private corner, removed from the curiosity of onlookers. There would be "no pressure to perform" and lots of mutual support. All agreed, seemingly enthusiastic. I booked a table. My chaperone Jean Martin and I arrived at the restaurant. We got to our reserved table, sat down and waited. And waited. And nobody showed up. Thus ended one of my larger lessons on social anxiety: My clients wouldn't say "no" to my face about a challenge that was just too steep.

As always, there's one more thing: Ordinary mortals have every right to make a hash of it. Professional performers don't. Stage actors mustn't fluff their lines, or they are out of a job. Trial lawyers mustn't fluff their summation, or trouble looms for their clients. Musicians must be in top form, or they'll end up poor. In the past, mediocre performers had a decent chance to get a gig. Since the appearance of the MP3 player, the money goes mostly to the best. There is no easy answer to a requirement for perfection. *In vivo exposure with paradoxical intent* won't work. There's no excuse when a professional reputation is at stake, unless a performer knows how to faint convincingly. *Imaginary exposure* (running a movie before one's inner eye) may help, also judiciously chosen medication. And a "plan B" might replace live performances with recordings.

Social phobics focus on the negative: Don't blush. Don't shake. Don't make a fool of yourself. It's impossible to prevent involuntary reactions like these. It's far better to focus on something positive instead, to aim for something you can make happen. Suppose you worry about being disliked. Turn your worry on its head. What can you do to be better liked? Ask yourself what you like people for. Is it for their brilliance and perfection? Is it for being considerate, light-hearted and easy going? Replacing "fears" by "wants" and "don'ts" with "dos" gives you more control. One "want" is experience from lots of practice, getting better by doing. Reputedly, Bernard Shaw conquered his fear of **public speaking** by stepping on a soapbox at every opportunity. He practiced, no matter what. He also had something to say, as did our Chair of Pathology in Heidelberg. I don't know if Doerr was ever nervous about public speaking. I only know that he practiced until he knew his lectures by heart. You could sometimes hear him shout them from the washroom. Here's a thought experiment for nervous speakers: What do you focus on in a speaker? Is it his appearance? (It might be, if he's outright cringeworthy.) Is it what he says and how he says it? To my mind, shaking like a leaf on stage won't matter half as much as making oneself easy to understand. A similar rule of thumb applies to meeting strangers at a party. The initial focus may be on appearances, but **conversation skills** can still make all the difference. Conversation is like a game of tennis (preferably without the competitiveness). You "serve" a question like "been to the film festival?" She may return your "serve" by commenting on a film. You put the ball back into her court with your own observations on the film. Or, if your "serve" wasn't returned, you ask a different question. Be ready with several topics. She-Who-Knows-these-things recommends researching the interests of new acquaintances for topics. Then you are girded for battle.

Some social phobics are excessively concerned with **the nether regions**. The *pee-shy syndrome* is one example. It befalls shy young men whose waterworks clam up in public washrooms. The sounds of a rich stream of urine splashing against the walls of a urinal might be overheard, and that's mortally embarrassing to an anxious mind. A medical student with this fear had to sit through a series of exams. Candidates were monitored even in the washroom, to ensure there was no cheating. The student understood the physiology of his condition. He prepared as best he could, avoiding caffeine and liquids to ease the urge. Still, there was no guarantee he wouldn't have to go, and this worried him to distraction. He couldn't concentrate and his test scores suffered. Treatment required *in vivo* exposure, joint visits to a public washroom. I prescribed a diuretic beforehand to ensure voiding, and off we went. - Neither one of us enjoyed these smelly visits, but they worked.

Below the belt lurks another fear that haunts men, the fear of being unable to "perform" in the sack. (Remember the minister in Gainesville.) It's usually worse with new partners and with demanding ones. Apologies for bluntness, but there's no such thing as being scared stiff. *"Psychogenic" impotence* (as opposed to impotence caused by a disease) results from **competitive in-**

hibition, an important principle in behavioral medicine. Sex is not a command performance. A fear of "failing" wins out over sexual arousal if it's intense enough, with unfortunate results. It's like the flow of saliva. Desire helps. Being carefree and relaxed helps. Trying harder doesn't. Either you feel keen and relaxed enough to enjoy yourself, or you don't. And if you don't, you "fail." One unfortunate fellow had the worst of it. Circumstances were unattractive to begin with at a red-light establishment. And to his partner, time was money. The balance between passion and distress was completely wrong, and passion failed to bloom.

Similar principles govern sexual response in women. Bad experiences can result in a hangover that lasts months and years, particularly after sexual violence and rape.

10. THE MANY FACES OF POSTTRAUMATIC STRESS DISORDER (PTSD)

After graduation from high school and a rather perfunctory medical examination, the German Army "invited" me to join the tank corps. Participation in a maneuver was on offer to whet my appetite. I wasn't keen, but why not enjoy the spectacle? The Army base was out there somewhere in the German countryside, and it was early in the morning. Soldiers were running about in camouflage uniforms and officers shouted commands over roaring engines. An officer lined me up with the other volunteers and assigned me to a tank of Korean War vintage. It had a big cannon, was deafeningly noisy inside, lacked upholstery and a decent suspension. You couldn't get a good view of the outside unless your head was sticking out of the driver's hatch, an unhealthy thing to do when the shooting starts. We rumbled out of the gate and into a large field with many humps and bumps. And then our tank broke down just as we crested a hill. It refused to move another inch and sat there, right in the line of "hostile" fire. We climbed out, sat in the grass and relaxed. Command declared us "technically dead." I liked the "technical" part and chose medical school over enlisting.

The experience didn't dampen my boyish curiosity about war and its machinery. Years later it led me onto the deck of a retired WWII US battleship (probably the USS North Carolina in Wilmington). Its grey superstructure was tall as houses and designed to withstand incoming fire. I stared in awe at cannons that could throw shells the size of small suitcases and wondered about the destruction they delivered. Shell shock came to mind without prompting. I also slid down the hatch of a WWII submarine. The world below was crowded with gauges, pipes and containers. The crew's bunks were ridiculously small and the place smelled of diesel. I wondered how any reasonable person could spend weeks and months in such narrow confines without going stark raving mad with claustrophobia. Remember the movie "Das Boot," the ping of hostile ASDIC and lethal charges exploding all around? War can be entertaining, provided you are not in it. Being in it is very different. The **war veterans** I examined in Gainesville and later in Toronto made this perfectly clear.

Below are a few of their stories.

A tail gunner suffered from persistent anxiety after WWII. He was flying home across the Channel after a bombing raid over Germany when cannon fire from a German fighter ripped through the fuselage of his bomber. It cut the intercom and communications ceased. The gunner was isolated in his perch in the tail of the bomber, as it drifted ever lower over the water, with engines running rough. He knew nothing about the health of pilot, the fate of fellow crewmembers and his chances of making it home. He got lucky. After a long, anxious wait the bomber cleared England's costal cliffs and belly-landed in a field near shore. He clambered out, shaken but physically unharmed. Soon afterwards, recurrent nightmares set in and intense claustrophobia. They troubled him for decades.

A Canadian Special Forces commando also suffered lasting psychological injury during WWII. His platoon surrounded a farmhouse during the battle of Monte Cassino. Tenacious German defenders were holding it. They refused to surrender and fought back for days, killing one of his men. Then they ran low on ammunition. Overwhelming firepower killed them. The commando returned home a silent man. He kept reliving the firefight and barely spoke for decades, except for essential utterances. He worked, but only by himself and in a menial capacity. Surprisingly he spoke to me at length. Even more surprising was his empathy for the German defenders. He broke down in tears as he described their courage and pointless death. He took some time to calm down.

A US veteran became severely anxious after surviving a surprise mortar attack on a medical facility in Vietnam. Unarmed soldiers scrambled for cover as mortars exploded amongst them in the middle of the night. Vietcong breached the perimeter and the base was on the verge of getting overrun. Help seemed far away. The attack was repelled, but it was a close call. The veteran felt on a hair trigger afterwards, jumpy and alert for noises in the night. He booby-trapped his Toronto flat against nighttime intruders, became suspicious of Asians and wouldn't enter parts of town where they lived. This seemed like paranoia, but it wasn't. He was open to reasoning and my presence eased his fear during visits to Asian communities in downtown Toronto. His defensive reflexes hadn't transitioned from wartime vigilance to the relaxed safety of the present. He remained hyper-alert, no matter how hard we tried to change this through exposure therapy

A Canadian Special Forces soldier retired from peacekeeping service after an RPG (rocket-propelled grenade) dealt his armored car a glancing blow. The car suffered only minimal damage. But the soldier's life took a downward turn afterwards for a combination of reasons. He became moody, irritable and slept poorly. One night he dozed off on the Toronto subway. Two subway employees "kicked him awake." He woke with a start, saw two strangers standing over him and "went ape." He was good at it. Both employees suffered substantial injuries. – His was in the only assault I have ever seen a war veteran commit. Charges were stayed after I submitted a letter in his defense.

The Canadian General *Romeo Dallaire* served as a peacekeeper through the horror of the Rwandan genocide. His memoir describes in detail its impact on his psychological health, his guilt and his long struggle with devastating memories. His book (10) is remarkably matter-of-fact. It moved me to tears. It also raises an important issue that comes up when a great wrong has been committed, when civility has been swept aside by an overwhelming disaster. Call it moral trauma (for "demoralizing"). Its victim has looked into the abyss and concluded that anything is possible and fighting back pointless. One **torture victim** exemplified this, a Somali refugee with a strikingly impassive attitude. He complained of pain and little else. It took a slow and gentle enquiry to get the rest. He had been arrested in his home country and forced to run behind a jeep with his hands tied to the vehicle until near death. Being let go came as a surprise to him. He must have expended considerable effort to reach safe haven, but he lacked plans beyond that and had no expectations for a better life. I believe his worldview had changed permanently to one of resignation and hopelessness, similar to the views of some concentration camp survivors.

Police offers are also not immune to PTSD. They get bitten by dogs, swarmed by crowds and have guns pointed at them. They see bloodied victims of traffic accidents and grisly murder scenes in their role of first responders and investigators, reminders of society's darker side and the many things that can go wrong. Traffic checks and walking the beat are harmless most of the time, but can turn dangerous at a moment's notice. Even healthy officers may display signs of hyper-vigilance. I met one for a restaurant lunch in a safe area of town. He seated himself with his back facing the wall. Sitting with his back facing the entrance "hadn't felt safe." Being the one to pull the trigger can also be very stressful. During a stakeout a SWAT officer had a dangerous suspect in in his sights. His order was to shoot in case of armed resistance. He felt reasonably confident that he was aiming at the right man, but visibility was poor. He wasn't as certain as he wanted to be. The crisis passed without a shot being fired, but his worries persisted. He became moody and developed persistent nightmares. Another SWAT officer had been reassigned to foot patrol for reasons unclear. A suspect drove a truck at him in a narrow alleyway late one evening, as if attempting to run him over. The officer pulled his weapon and aimed. He didn't fire, but faced an "internal" review and a potential reprimand for drawing his weapon "prematurely." Disciplinary action was stayed after his psychological state received due consideration. Officers like him may feel misunderstood and abandoned by the Force. They have few confidantes to discuss their experiences with and few opportunities for "reality checks" with persons from outside the force. It's no wonder then that an attitude of "us versus them" develops easily amongst some of them.

Frightening illness can also leave deep emotional scars, as does **rape**. Anything that impedes breath may cause panic, chest pain during a heart attack and severe asthma, also man-made horrors like waterboarding. Choking during a rape is simply terrifying. The victim can't breathe. She doesn't know when the chokehold will be released. She fears for her life and her only hope is mercy. The aftermath brings more fear: If it happened once, it can happen again. Dating feels like recklessness. Precautions are never are quite enough. She may tell a friend about her whereabouts and whom she'll be with. She may avoid alcohol consumption, drinks of unknown provenance, abandoned parking garages and deserted streets. Precautions improve her odds and guarantee nothing. Any man she meets may be another wolf in sheep's clothing. It's impossible to tell a potential assailant from a genuine friend until it is too late. That's true particularly for acquaintance rape, rape by a trusted person. Some rape survivors deal with this combination of ambiguity and fear by ignoring risk altogether. There's one clue though that should never be ignored. *If a date seems controlling, domineering, potentially jealous* *and coercive, beware! You don't want him to "own" you* in the way a jealous husband "owned" his wife. He stabbed her to death while shouting "you are mine" (evidence from a murder trial). The serial killer Paul Bernardo also "owned" his victims, combining extreme sexual domination with murder (see below).

Examples of PTSD raise important questions. What exactly is "trauma?" What kind of stress will cause it? What are the signs? Who is most vulnerable? "Trauma" is a term that's often used without definition. Casual use hollows out its meaning. Psychological trauma results from an overwhelming experience, one that's beyond the victims ability to cope. It's disruptive. It alters the victim's physiological and mental state. It alters the trajectory of her life, turns hope into fear and despair, good prospects into lowly subsistence. To what extent can a recovery take place? I had asked myself these questions many times. And now I had to answer them for the Courts, when the German Consulate General in Toronto retained me to assess the claims of Jewish concentration camp survivors against the German State.

11. THE HORROR OF NAZI CONCENTRATION CAMPS

The Nazi concentration camps embody racism in its most organized and lethal form. Their construction began in 1933 after Hitler came to power. One of the first was Dachau near Munich, followed by some sixty-seven others. Initially the camps housed dissidents, gays and gypsies (the Roma). Then Jews were deported there in ever increasing numbers under the guise of re-settlement in conquered territories. In 1942 the SS leader Heydrich convened a meeting of senior Nazi officials at the Wannseekonferenz in a palais near a lake in Berlin. The palais is now a museum commemorating the Holocaust. Senior Nazi officials organized details there for the "final solution" to the "Jewish question". The Jews of Europe would be rounded up, confined to camps, forced into hard labor and ultimately "exterminated."

An estimated six million Jews succumbed to the camps, to exhaustion, illness, starvation, shooting and poison gas in purpose-built chambers. Eleven million non-Jews also died in the camps according to the Washington Holocaust Museum. The deportees were taken there in locked cattle cars, often without heat, food or water. Many did not survive the journey.

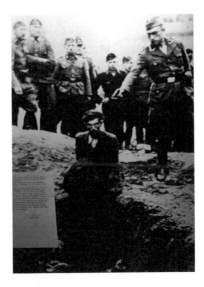

An execution; from the Holocaust Museum, Munich

All this is widely known and sometimes denied. The film "Schindler's List" reminds us of the horrors of camp Krakow-Plaszow in credible detail (as survivors from this camp told me). Auschwitz/Birkenau may have been worse. Upon arrival at the train station there, detainees were "selected" for slave labor under the cynical motto of *"Arbeit macht frei"* (work sets you free) or sent directly to their death in the gas chambers. Those who survived the selection were tattooed with an identification number beginning with an "A" (resembling a triangle) on the volar side of their left forearm. Some underwent potentially deadly medical experiments under the direction of Dr. Mengele, a sadistic Nazi doctor who tested the extreme limits of human endurance. Near the end of the War many detainees succumbed while driven west by retreating German forces. Small memorials dot the contemporary German countryside to commemorate these death marches.

After the War the Allies confronted the German public with the realities of the holocaust and a "collective guilt" that was not easily forgiven. Villagers who lived near former camps were confronted with the evidence. School children (including myself) watched footage from Auschwitz that was taken shortly after liberation. Footage included gas chambers, barracks with impossibly crowded sleeping quarters, dazed survivors looking skeletal in striped uniforms and corpses piled high. In the early Fifties the German *Bundestag* (Parliament) passed several laws for restitution (*Wiedergutmachung*). One law restored stolen property to its original owners. Another onr compensated Jewish survivors for medical and psychological damages sustained in the camps. The law transferred the usual burden of proof from plaintiff to defendant. Anyone who had been in a KZ for one year or more was presumed to suffer from significant psychological trauma. Applications would succeed unless the State disproved this premise. Compensation depended on the severity of a claimant's current symptoms, his (hypothetical) vocational potential at the time of incarceration, the impact racist persecution had on it and the resulting trajectory of his life. Many claimants had moved overseas by the time the law came into effect. They could still apply, if they had credible documentation of their incarceration and its duration. Overseas physicians retained by the German State provided the medical assessments and German Courts adjudicated the matter.

In the late Seventies, a fellow staff member from the Department of Obstetrics and Gynecology at St. Mike's (Charles Luttor) contacted me on behalf of the Courts: Would I be willing to provide the necessary psychiatric assessments of concentration camp (*KZ*) survivors? Court files were in German, my mother tongue. They would provide proof of *KZ* stay and its duration, and that would take care of the "ticklish" burden of proof as far as Nazi persecution was concerned. Only the nature of claimants' symptoms, their severity and their impact on work and career development needed to be assessed. Government would provide me with medico-legal "guidelines" for the assessments according to compensation law. I would be function as a "Friend of the Court," be accredited in Frankfurt, Munich and Berlin (later also Vienna) and receive a modest fee for each case. Court appearances would not be required. Charles Luttor provided such assessments in his specialty. The interviews were "difficult" even for him with his Hungarian heritage. They would be particularly difficult for someone with a German name tainted by Nazi guilt.

My first applicant arrived at St. Mike's with a paralegal in tow. The paralegal deposited his briefcase on my desk with a laud crash and began to quiz me on my knowledge of the holocaust. I was getting my first taste of an adversarial situation. After hearing him out, answering his questions and accepting supporting documentation I relegated him to the waiting room. The claimant then cooperated. I took me a long time over the next few days to write up my first report.

Getting quizzed about the holocaust was perfectly acceptable, especially in a medico-legal context and at a time when ongoing holocaust denials added insult to injury. I was prepared for that. I was familiar with footage from the camps since school and had spoken with my dad about the holocaust and his chance encounter with an execution squad. At university I had been a member of a German-Jewish friendship group. In Sweden, I had met a Jewish student from Poland who described how the holocaust had surprised her family. Feeling an affinity to German culture and science, they had refused to see the threat. But the role as assessor was new to me. I came to realize that I was not just a doctor taking a history. My role made me a representative of the nation that had committed these atrocities.

Assessors have feelings too, just like everybody else. I harbored guilt and shame for "being German." Other nations had also committed atrocities. But the Nazi camps were as bad as can be, and two wrongs don't make a right. It's been suggested that certain cultural traits enabled German atrocities. Was this true and did I harbor these? I had learned as a child and later as a student to resent the wanton exercise of power. It took me longer to question the indifference, the unquestioning loyalties and subservience that enabled the holocaust. My only defense was the accident of birth. None of us choose our ethnicity and how we are raised, not Jews, not Germans, not anyone else. Conduct deserves scrutiny, ethnicity never. And that wasn't all. I also had to guard against my anger at being accused of something I hadn't done, anger that could bias me against a claimant. I had to guard equally against the opposite, against favoring claimants out of guilt, pity and in the absence of supporting evidence. I needed to develop an assessment protocol that excluded bias, and in a hurry. This may sound unfeeling, but the alternative would have been opinion based on emotion instead of fact. Sleepless nights drove home this point.

I started out with associative interviewing and projective psychological testing, notably the house-tree-person test. The drawings illustrated the barren worldview of the survivors, leafless trees with broken branches, houses with shuttered windows and stick-like little people that stood in the middle of nowhere. They captured emotions well, but were useless as a quantitative measure of symptom severity and disability. Fortunately, my recently acquired research skills came to the rescue. An improved assessment protocol included psychological tests that were accepted internationally and could be scored quantitatively. A semi-structured interview with predetermined questions added diagnostic reliability. I developed an assessment protocol and followed it consistently. This made assessments more elaborate than the Courts required, but also better. By the end of my appointment, I had assessed over five hundred survivors over the course of three decades. Their stories changed me, my beliefs and expectations. If the holocaust happened once, it can happen again. Persistent racism of many stripes, slavery, ethnic cleansing, the remnants of Stalin's Gulag, the Khmer Rouge's killing fields, "re-education" camps for the

Uighurs, ISIS, the Rwandan genocide and the cruelties of residential schools for native children make this likely, particularly if we naively believe that the Holocaust was something only Hitler's Nazis are capable of perpetrating.

The survivors had haunting stories to tell. Near starvation was the rule in the camps. The "capo system" coopted inmates into supervisory roles and enforcers of camp discipline. (For details on Stalin's similar system read Anne Appelbaum's book (11) on the USSR's "Gulag. Food rations improved with good "service" and resulted in crippling survivor's guilt over collaboration with the enemy, most strikingly in one man who had been ordered to pull gold teeth from the skulls of the dead right outside the gas chamber. Others collected hair and clothing from these victims. Inmates were crowded into unheated facilities and stacked on bunks like cords of wood. An Allied bombing raid on a munitions factory near Auschwitz added to their troubles. Survival required incredible hardiness and self-control. I wonder if this second "selection" led to the remarkable uniformity amongst the survivors I saw. Most were small, bent by age, reticent, polite, tense and really, really tough. They also were model citizens. I uncovered not a single case of substance use (which disproves claims that substance use is an integral part of PTSD). None smoked and few drank much coffee. Most were irritable, but none were violent. Almost all worked hard in menial occupations and lived in near poverty. Their complaints were very similar. Terrifying nightmares were their most prominent feature. They disrupted sleep to the point of sleep deprivation, in itself a health hazard. Most of them experienced chronic depression, irritability, persistent anxiety, a fear of strangers in uniform and had a gloomy outlook.

The assessments were not conducted with later publication in mind. An analysis of data was conducted years later on the urgings of colleagues. Eventually I published a first set of findings on one-hundred-and twenty-four survivors with the psychologist Brian Cox and a second one on three-hundred-and-fifty with the psychologist Neil Rector from CAMH.

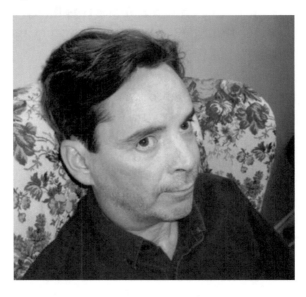

Brian Cox, psychologist and researcher

Both publications compared tattooed *Auschwitz* survivors with survivors from other camps, including *Stuthof, Bergen-Belsen, Plaszow, Dachau* and *Buchenwald*. Both have been widely cited in the scientific literature. The first one found that tattooed Auschwitz survivors were more impaired than the survivors from other camps. It also contained more first claims than the second study. The second study could not replicate this difference between camps. Both studies revealed an almost identical pattern of symptoms characteristic for severe PTSD, with terrifyingly vivid dreams and memories that came unbidden and made survivors feel as if their horrors were happening all over again, day after day and night after night.

The Nazi concentration camps destroyed millions of innocent lives. Only the accident of birth had put them in harm's way, nothing else. What enabled this mass murder of innocents in a country famous for its philosophers and thinkers? Did a rabid form of nationalism ally itself with long-standing anti-Semitism and anti-science to spawn a system this vile? Historians and sociologists are better placed to answer this question than myself. I just ask a contemporary one: How can we be so sure that the enablers of the Holocaust, prejudice, hatred and blinkered determination, were a uniquely German problem, unlikely to rise again, this after the destabilizing "big lie" about a stolen election that would have made Dr. Goebbels proud? The Holocaust didn't begin the moment Hitler came to power. It began gradually over eight years and under the guise of good intentions.

12.THE MISERY OF CHRONIC PAIN

I must have been a glutton for punishment when adding chronic pain to my caseload. But, as Oscar Wilde put it so nicely, "I can resist anything but temptation." I couldn't resist when the surgeon Ray Evans invited me to join the Smythe Pain Clinic at Toronto General Hospital. Ray had founded it and made it the first multi-disciplinary pain clinic in Canada. Its original mandate was cancer pain. Then its focus widened to include chronic pain, the pain that refuses to go away, is all over your body, lacks a demonstrable cause and slowly but surely ruins your life.

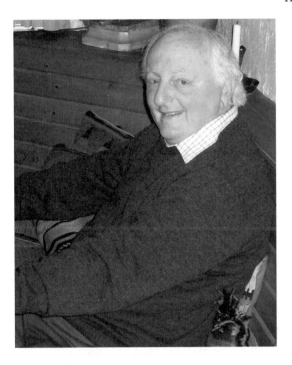

Ray Evans, surgeon and director of the Smythe Pain Clinic

The Smythe Pain Clinic had an arrangement that was novel at the time. It combined surgery, neurology, anesthesia and psychiatry under one roof. It also combined everything we knew about a patient in one single chart, seemingly a small administrative feature, in reality a groundbreaking change that saved our patients from the "medical runaround" (8). A "runaround" can happen when one busy specialist refers a puzzling case to another busy specialist. He sees the patient in a less than timely fashion, writes up an opinion without firm conclusions, then refers the patient back to the first doctor or to a third for further examination. And when of them drops the ball, the runaround gets maddening. In the Pain Clinic, the ball stayed put. Instead of sending letters by snail mail, we knocked on a door down the hallway or slid a piece of paper under it if something needed discussing. Occasionally, Ray the surgeon and I the psychiatrist also examined patients jointly.

Chronic pain is misery plain and simple. There are no smiles. It's "pain all over" that never lets up. Analgesics don't seem to work and nothing tells you what to do next. Accidents can start a slide into chronic pain, but they don't explain it and why this happens to some but not to others. Pain can be "idiopathic," without apparent cause and without any outward signs. Many sufferers appear outwardly healthy, and tempers flare when they feel silently accused of exaggeration. Contested compensation claims add more irritation. Fortunately, this may be changing. A systematic review of the scientific literature has confirmed chronic pain as a valid diagnostic entity (see below). Treatable sub-types are also emerging. Rheumatologists now recognize *polymyalgia rheumatica* as a distinct pain disorder that may respond to potent anti-inflammatories. *Fibromyalgia* remains part of the chronic pain puzzle last time I looked.

I had a lot to learn when I joined the Pain Clinic. I participated in surgical examinations, picked neurologists' brains and learned about nerve blocks from Connie Bubela, our anesthesiologist. Ray, the head of the clinic, spent long evenings entering patient data into a database on his own time. It was a labor of love that enabled statistical evaluation. Statistics disposed of prejudicial "diagnoses" like the "Mediterranean back," a false belief about a tendency to "dramatize" in people with a Southern origin. They revealed important commonalities between pain patients with and without a prior history of accidents and the interaction between anxiety, depression and pain (see below). Our neurologist Peter Watson published a study on treating *postherpetic neuralgia* with amitriptyline, a "first" in the field. And the TGH pharmacy maintained a separate database on *adverse drug reactions* and *drug-on-drug interactions*, vital to the understanding of failing drug therapy. Interesting as all this was, it still begged the question of how a psychiatrist could contribute to the clinical management of pain. Patients insist that pain isn't "all in their mind." "Pain is pain" is how the psychiatrist Howard Merskey summed up their plight. **Living with pain** is more complex however. It's an interaction between pain perception, neurophysiology and external conditions, that needs to be examined from several points of view. - It was my point of entry.

To lay people, pain is as straightforward as a phone call: An injury sends a warning signal along a sensory nerve path to the spinal column and from there to the brain. The signal includes details about quality (burning, tearing, nagging), severity and location. That's only half the story. The other half is just as important. Two **feedback loops** regulate incoming pain signals. Ronald Melzack's *"gate theory"* represents the first: Incoming pain signals have to pass through a "gate" before they reach the brain. This "gate" can turn down severity, just like a volume control turns down a noisy stereo. The neurosurgeon Ron Tasker based a *"dorsal column stimulator"* on Melzack's theory. It's implanted on the spinal cord and produces a mild electric current at the push of a button. The current competes with the pain signal and closes Melzack's "gate." A second feedback loop involves *endorphin*, the body's own pain reliever. Pain triggers endorphin release and that in turn dampens pain severity and distress. Concomitant excitement and exertion may trigger a greater release, which may explain the peculiar lack of pain soldiers and athletes may experience in the immediate aftermath of injury.

This much about neurophysiology; now to the treatment of **the "whole person:"** Some patients fight several problems all at once, a second illness or a lot of stress. In legal lingo, they are the *"thin-skulled clients,"* the vulnerable ones who are ill-equipped to control the impact of pain on their daily lives. They are travelling a bumpy road already, and pain upsets their proverbial apple cart more thoroughly than it would under easier conditions. Could I help these people? I couldn't rid them of the pain they felt. That had been tried by the time they consulted me. But I could practice **damage control** and reduce the impact of pain on their daily lives. I prescribed antidepressants to relieve sleeplessness and depression. I reviewed drug side effects like constipation, sedation and poor memory and suggested remedies. I educated patients on the *half-life* of analgesics and the *break-through pain* that may develop after a major portion of an analgesic has left the bloodstream. And I did whatever I could to simplify prescriptions. For that, I asked every new client to present all pills for inspection, including herbal remedies. Ten different prescriptions were pretty much the rule. More wasn't unusual. One standout turned up with two full shopping bags. He took his pills according to the way he felt on any given day, risking all kinds of side effects. He had blue-pill days, yellow-pill and red-pill days, but no no-pill days.

Several factors account for such **polypharmacy** (multiple and potentially incompatible prescriptions). Many patients continue taking medications that should have been discontinued when new ones were prescribed. Maybe the doctor "forgot," maybe the patient wanted to hang on to them, just in case. When only one doctor prescribes and only one pharmacy fills the script, polypharmacy is easier to prevent than when one hand doesn't know what the other one is doing. And there's more. Excruciating pain is impossible to ignore. The doctor can't just "sit back and do nothing." She must "do something," prescribe physiotherapy or a nice spa (a popular remedy in Europe). If this doesn't do the trick, she may feel pressured to prescribe a stronger analgesic. Saying "no" to that is hard. Discontinuing a painkiller is even harder, for reason described below. I never got anyone off opiates. It wasn't a total loss though. Most of my habitués ended up with fewer meds and fewer side effects, a small victory of sorts.

Fewer opiates are nowadays prescribed than in the recent past. Renewed caution has swung the proverbial pendulum away from opiate over-use in chronic pain and minor injury. That's fair enough, unless the pendulum over-shoots into the under-medication of cancer pain and post-surgical pain that existed in the past, based on an unfounded fear of addiction. Bringing the pendulum to a halt somewhere near an evidence-based middle will require cool heads and diagnostic rigor, lest we end up parsing opioids where they are badly needed. I would also love to see an end to the uncritical advertisement of analgesics on TV. It's malpractice by media. Analgesics aren't soap powder, and glowing testimonials by "real patients" can be misleading. They don't ask the necessary questions about the balance between risk and benefit. They also don't suggest that pain can get better without drugs, sometimes by waiting just a little.

Years ago, the psychologist Wilbur Fordyce was looking for a new way to understand chronic pain. An observer can't see a patient's pain (unless she monitors "evoked potentials" on an EEG or changes on a PET scan). But she can see "**pain behavior**" (pain-induced behavior change). She can also observe the **consequences of pain behavior**. A thought experiment may illustrate the usefulness of this concept. Suppose a hiker pulls a muscle while out on a trail. She has two basic choices. She can quit, and she can keep on hiking. Lets assume she keeps on hiking. Suppose a second hiker also pulls a muscle. Let's assume he quits and catches a ride home. Why do the two hikers behave so differently? Is his pain more severe than hers when his injury is not? We don't know that. Chances are that the second hiker worried more about his injury than the first, and that's why he quit. According to Fordyce, his expectations were more pessimistic. He "suffered" more. And that matters, because he risks getting flabby and unfit as a consequence. If his doctor assures him that moderate exercise is harmless, even essential, that physiotherapy can help even when it hurts, he may reverse course, go back to hiking and staying fit. In short, **worry and expectations alter pain behavior**. And doctors need to manage that.

Fordyce's pain clinic in Oregon eased opiate withdrawal according to the same principle: Most opioid users expect substantial discomfort after dose-reduction. That's correct of course, but only within limits. Besides dose-reduction, expectations also play a role. The Oregon program dealt with this **placebo effect** by reducing daily doses "blindly," with prior consent. Identical quantities of syrup disguised the opioid dose dissolved in them. The participants didn't know how much they were taking on each given day. Nor did they know how worried they should be at each step in the withdrawal process.

And there's still more to know.

We can't **measure pain** directly and that's a huge disadvantage. We are flying blind unless we trace its peaks and valleys. Fortunately, we can measure pain behavior. We can also measure the severity of **complaints**. The Smythe Pain Clinic did this by handing out questionnaires and psychometrics. We asked our patients to indicate painful areas by darkening them on a human silhouette with a pen. That gave us pain location and extent. We asked them to add an estimate of severity (0-10). We also asked about the impact of pain on sleep, about what eased the pain and what made it worse. I added questions about pain frequency (the percentage of waking hours spent in pain), about anxiety, depression and the impact of pain on daily activities. Why ask all these questions?

Mood is the lens through which we view reality. When we feel happy, expectations are rosy and we cope better. When we feel anxious and low, we expect the worst and act accordingly. Analysis of research data revealed that *continuous pain* correlated with *depressed mood.* And depressed mood (but not anxiety) correlated with *greater impact of pain on daily living.* In other words, when people feel down, they act the part, and vice versa. They cope less well, are less active physically, socially and vocationally. And when they hit bottom, they may lose their job and suffer economic hardship. That's the "perfect storm" that damage control and a permissive **work environment** hope to prevent.

When I was a medical student some rotter threw me off the mat in judo. My neck became stiff and sore. An orthopedic surgeon diagnosed a hairline fracture at a cervical vertebra, prescribed a restraining collar and rest. I followed his advice and got better. This wasn't the end of it. My neck pain recurred and one arm became partially paralyzed. The paralysis resolved and pain improved. But it kept recurring, each episode lasting from months to years. Painkillers and muscle relaxants were useless and I stopped them. Traction seemed to help. I took my portable traction unit to work during severe episodes and scheduled breaks for its use. This kept the worst spasms at bay and helped me maintain an almost undiminished work schedule. My point is this: I couldn't have maintained my output on a job that didn't permit breaks. "**Disablement**" (as occupational therapists call this process) occurs when rigid working conditions prevent you from "listening to your body" and taking necessary breaks. When you then lose your job, you lose endurance and work skills. With the passage of time, your chances for successful rehabilitation decline. And that completes the process of disablement.

Chronic pain has wheels within wheels, visible only to the inquisitive eye. To get your proverbial arms around it you need to evaluate it without prejudice, practice damage control, maintain work skills and fitness, be patient and let the pain burn itself out. Preserving sleep, keeping a positive outlook and staying active are crucially important. Help from employers can make a big difference, as an exhaustive review of pain studies has demonstrated. It may right the ship even in a perfect storm.

13.WHY THE FUSS ABOUT SCIENCE?

"**S**cience is just another opinion and it's often wrong." My blood pressure rose when I heard this at a party. I took the bait, failing to realize that I was charging a well-entrenched position: "Science isn't an opinion. It's a method of enquiry," I lectured. "And it's usually right." This didn't cut any ice. It would have been wiser to ask the good man how he arrived at his opinion, then challenge him to prove his point.

Modern living would be impossible without the benefits of science. You can enjoy it though without knowing much about it. Most of us don't look under the hood of our car. We just drive it. But when something goes wrong, when something needs fixing, knowing how it works does help. Here's my point: Prescription drugs, vaccines and public health directives are the same in this regard as cars. When something gets controversial as now with healthcare directives and the pandemic, knowing how to tell good advice from bad and science from junk science is miles better than believing what somebody tells you. That's particularly important when you don't know who this somebody might be. Without basic science knowledge and credible sources, an informed debate about health care is dead in the water. Quackery and the "health scare of the day" get undue attention. "Opinion makers" get away with outrageous claims. And a public that doesn't understands the reasoning behind health care advisories is less likely to follow them.

Unfortunately, research about pandemics, vaccines and prescription drugs happens largely out of sight from the very public it's meant to protect. The following offers a primer and a look behind the scenes.

According to the US Department of Health, total US health care spending reached 3.3 trillion dollars in 2018; that's $ 11,172 per capita and rising. Is it money well spent? That's an open question. We try out a new car before we buy. We do less with patent medicines. Fortunately, we try vaccines and prescription drugs very vigorously. The public needs to know how that's done. That's far better than blind faith and easier to understand than you might think. You probably know most of the methodology already and use it at work. Why not use it for a critical reading of health care news?

Take **market research**. It polls prospective customers for characteristics like age, ability and interests (read medical diagnostics), then designs its product accordingly (read drug and vaccine development). It analyses sales (read drug study) and asks if product changes improved sales **significantly**, or if improvement came about by nothing more than **chance**. On the stock market, we don't want greed and fear to **bias** our trades. We use **objective metrics** instead (read description and quantitative measures). When we borrow money, we guard against compound interest, to safeguard our financial prospects against spiraling debt (read virus epidemiology). We don't fall for poor odds (read **probability**) at the casino. We don't fall for the "gambler's fallacy" either by confusing a **random** process like rolling the dice with predictable **averages** that will kick in if we only gamble long enough. As travelers, we consider **risk** from COVID infection before we leave home (read epidemiology). The absolute number of currently COVID-infected people per day, month or year (**prevalence**) at our destination tells us a little about that. **Prevalence rates** tell us a lot more, by indicating the **proportion** of infected persons per million. How much protection does vaccination afford? Proportionate numbers must be used there as well, to avoid an error called **base-rate fallacy**. Omitting the crucial fact that a large number of vaccinated people may yield as many hospitalizations as a much smaller number of unvaccinated people would create the false impression that vaccination is pointless and a piece of dangerous misinformation (Newscasters, are you listening?). We also mustn't be fooled by glowing reports that crop one axis on a graph to make a small change look desirably large (12). None of this is out of reach for the non-statistician and help is near from books like "Statistics Without Tears" (13). Add to this the rule of cross-checking dubious information of unknown provenance with information that comes from multiple more credible sources, and you'll be well on your way to being street-proofed.

Now to the pills you swallow and the jabs you take:

Prescription drugs and vaccines have to pass strict reviews before their release to pharmacies. First come **safety experiments** with laboratory animals, then experiments with healthy volunteers. These are followed by an **"open label trial"** with patient-volunteers (similar to my biofeedback trial) and finally by a **controlled trial** with another set of patient-volunteers (see below). The process is as tedious and expensive as it sounds, but indispensable. It starts out with the "**null hypothesis**," the assumption that the drug's no good. The drug trial has to disprove this assumption. It has to accomplish this by following a protocol that excludes placebo effects and bias, also by conducting a data analysis that uses accepted statistical methods. It must be stringent with its interpretation of these data and conclude from them only what they support. Only after that's done and dusted can the drug maker submit its drug to the FDA, to Canada Health, the EU Medicines Agency and the UK Health and Medicines Agency for approval, which is far from automatic.

Now to the way this works in real life.

14.THERE REALLY
IS A KALAMAZOO

In the late Eighties, the American Food And Drug Administration (FDA) and Health Canada required a placebo-controlled treatment study before releasing Xanax as a prescription drug for the treatment of panic disorder and agoraphobia. An earlier study had suggested such benefits from the antidepressant Imipramine. Open-label (uncontrolled pilot) studies had suggested the same for Xanax, but more rapidly and with fewer side effects than with Imipramine. Upjohn, the maker of Xanax, was looking for a co-investigator. Participation in the study offered hands-on training in objective assessment methods and an opportunity to learn from accomplished colleagues. I jumped at it, this in spite of my preference for behavior therapy. Thus began one of the most exciting times in my professional life.

"There really is a Kalamazoo" asserted a T-shirt when I arrived at the local airport. Some fifteen other researchers also arrived there from Boston, New York, Montreal, Charleston and Toronto. Upjohn had taken great care to organize the trial and attract the necessary talent. The company owned a large property in the countryside near the Kellogg Forest, more resort than industrial site. It became the setting for our first meeting, with many more to come later on in Boston, New York, Zurich, London and Vienna, for this and for other trials. The Kalamazoo site included sleeping quarters, conference rooms and a gym, a dining room with top chefs, a book of recipes as a take-home gift and a well-stocked wine cellar. Ponds on the property teemed with trout, and fishing rods sat waiting against pond-side benches for the likes of me, or so I thought. There was no time for fishing. Up-john-issue alarm clocks summoned us at six every morning for training sessions that lasted the entire day. Lunch was a hurried affair. Dinner however was sumptuous, offered time to compare notes, swap stories and find light relief.

I am most grateful to Jim Ballenger, Chair then of the North Carolina department, for his instructions on the use of beer bottle caps as Frisbees.

To qualify for the study, volunteers had to meet specific **entrance criteria**. They had to experience "panic anxiety" (the frights, if you ask me) at least once per week, this for statistical reasons. They had to discontinue all medications two weeks before the actual trial and remain free of caffeine and alcohol. The treatment part of the trial employed a classical **double-blind placebo-controlled design**: Neither the volunteers nor the assessors knew who was taking Xanax and who was taking the fake pill (the placebo). Allocation to drug versus placebo was randomized by computer-generated roster, to prevent a biased selection of volunteers. Going forward, periodic assessments would then evaluate volunteers' mood, anxiety, agoraphobic restrictions and drug side effects during treatment.

The investigators rehearsed the use of all assessment instruments in a series of training sessions before the start of the trial. Training included the rating of videotaped patient interviews with psychometrics and a standardized clinical interview, the SCID (structured clinical interview according to DSM). The SCID was pre-recorded and had to be read from a page, question after question, to improve **diagnostic reliability**. All of us were experienced clinicians, accustomed to asking questions according to our own judgment. The SCID did not allow this. It was a necessary evil. Without the SCID, variations between interviewers' questions would produce a "noisy" (read inaccurate) variety of answers. This would happen because a question was asked differently, not because the interviewee was experiencing different symptoms. Too many "apples" would then be mislabeled for "oranges," and that would jeopardize the diagnostic reliability essential to clinical research.

After a week of rehearsals and brainstorming I returned to Toronto, tired but elated. A second set of training sessions followed at Massachusetts General Hospital with live patient-volunteers, a third at the Allan Memorial in Montreal (in connection with a different drug trial). The training sessions proved invaluable to my own research and for medico-legal purposes, less so for clinical interviewing where nuance and ad hoc adjustments matter more than agreement between interviewers.

Drug research is stressful, to put it mildly. Success promises career-advancing publications to investigators and large financial rewards to the drug maker. Failure means major losses to all involved. That showed as the trial date approached. The pressure rose on corporate staff, on the investigators and the roving "QUATs," the members of external quality assessment teams who made sure that investigators followed every rule. Before the trial, investigators had to recruit the statistically required number of patient-volunteers and keep them from dropping out over the course of the trial, a vital exercise as insufficient numbers would jeopardize statistical reliability and sink the trial. Investigators were available to the volunteers 24/7. They answered their questions and distress calls without doing anything that would break protocol. It was quite a balancing act. The "QUAT squads" from Upjohn and the FDA dropped in unannounced, pulled files, reviewed procedures and scrutinized data. Some visits felt like the FBI was coming to town. Once the clinical part of the trial was finished, statisticians crunched the numbers for reliability and levels of significance. Thereafter, lead investigators wrote it all up and submitted their manuscripts for peer review to scientific journals. After that was done, the FDA and the Canadian Departments of Health conducted their own review. And then, and only then, could medical practitioners prescribe the drug.

Fortunately, there were some lighter moments.

One volunteer phoned in a state of high anxiety. Both of her legs had "turned blue." Xanax turning legs blue? Would it be "pulled" and re-examined for toxicity before our trial could be resumed? Disaster loomed and telephone wires were running hot between Toronto, Boston and Kalamazoo. Then the truth emerged: Our volunteer had bought a new pair of blue jeans. She wanted them to fit good and tight. So she pulled them on and sat in a hot bath to make them shrink. And that caused the dye to leach onto the skin of her legs. - An international sigh of relief followed this revelation.

Our share of **the first Xanax trial** (in a series of three) took place at Toronto General Hospital (TGH). Headquarters were at Massachusetts General Hospital. Ad hoc conferences were held with little notice in New York, requiring that we drop everything and hop on a flight. Carefully planned schedules crumbled. Leisure times vanished. And sleep turned restless. I flagged down a private car at LaGuardia airport once to get to a meeting in time. Fortunately, we had lots of support. Earlier my friend and colleague Richard Swinson and I had launched the Anxiety Disorders Clinic at TGH. Without a helpful staff that covered emergencies, without patients that were very patient indeed and without tolerant spouses, participation in the trial would have been very difficult. The media also helped. Potential volunteers were understandably hesitant and had many questions. After a press release and a few TV interviews, they just wanted to join, few questions asked. This was convenient, but also a cautionary tale. Seeing something advertised on TV can be more convincing than a face-to-face interview with the same doctor.

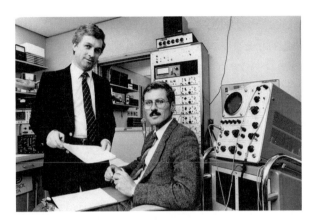

Richard Swinson (left) and the author opening the
Anxiety Disorders Clinic at TGH; Getty Images

Now to the **results**: Anxiety and depression have a biological basis. Twin studies and genetic research indicate this. But there's more to it than that. "Biological" doesn't equal "needing medication." Panickers (people with the frights) can get better without drugs. During the two-week "washout period" before the actual Xanax trial (time spent without meds, alcohol and caffeine), almost one-quarter of our volunteers got better to such an extent, they no longer qualified for the trial. What had happened? Emotional support and explanations of the nature of panic anxiety may have helped. **Abstention from alcohol and caffeine** may have helped some more, a phenomenon I noted earlier when describing my own frights on a plane.

Upon completion of the trial, data analysis compared Xanax with placebo (the fake drug). Panic frequency was the main outcome criterion. Our volunteers had improved "significantly" (in statistical terms) and remained improved for as long as they were taking Xanax. This looked like a break-through, convincing enough to alter my clinical management of panic disorder. Then doubts developed. How would patients fare that weren't as diagnostically "pure" as our study volunteers? And how would they fare after they had stopped the drug?

Most family doctors will confirm that many of their patients have more than one problem. This raises an important question. Can the results from a "pure" sample with only one well-defined illness predict what happens with patients that suffer simultaneously from illnesses like asthma, from stress and social problems? Questions from skeptical GPs reinforced my doubts. The British psychiatrist Isaac Marks agreed. He'd "love to do a trial with volunteers who had failed entrance criteria," to see to what extent our findings could be applied to a more naturalistic setting. – We didn't get the chance.

A second Xanax trial at the Toronto and Montreal sites examined the second question, how patients would manage after Xanax was withdrawn. Results from a **withdrawal study** were as discouraging as the first study was encouraging. All our volunteers completed their withdrawal. That was the good news. It meant they weren't hopelessly addicted to Xanax. Now to the bad news: Every one of them relapsed shortly after withdrawal. Some were worse off than before. To their credit, Upjohn agreed to fund **a third Xanax** trial. It was complex, to say the least. It compared Xanax with therapist-assisted exposure therapy (behavior therapy), separately and in combination, before and after Xanax withdrawal. The trial became known as **the London-Toronto study**. It was (and probably still is) the largest and the most comprehensive trial on the treatment of panic anxiety and agoraphobia. It included six-months of follow-up without any treatment, an aspect that yielded important long-term outcome data.

Study design was again of the classical double-blind placebo-controlled variety, more demanding even than for the first two trials. This time, compared four different treatment combinations with each other. The (real) *behavioral treatment* was therapist-assisted exposure therapy in feared situations (remember the Florida lady). The *fake behavioral treatment* was relaxation training. The real drug treatment was *Xanax.* And the fake drug treatment (the *placebo*) contained no active ingredient. Treatments and fake treatments were combined four different ways to form *four sub-groups* of randomly selected volunteers, to determine what treatment worked best. A six-month long follow-up without further treatment was added by the end of the active trial, to demonstrate lasting outcome, the ultimate proof of the pudding.

Our **results** were unpopular with Upjohn. *Behavior therapy alone was better than Xanax alone. It was also better alone than in combination with Xanax. In addition, it produced slow but persistent improvement that continued during six months of treatment-free follow-up.* As in the two preceding studies, volunteers on Xanax (Alprazolam) improved first and relapsed later as Xanax was withdrawn. Relaxation training also did not help.

Our findings were aired in the august setting of Geneva conference rooms and generated a lot of heat. I am unaware of any subsequent support from Upjohn to disseminate these results. But published they were after additional funding for data analysis was obtained through London University in the UK. A subsequent exchange of Letters to the Editor in the British Journal of Psychiatry documents a controversy that continued for some time. I signed one of the letters authored by Isaac Marks, the British lead investigator for the London-Toronto study and a highly respected researcher. It is dry and to the point: "Scientific research and drug marketing are two separate disciplines." They should not be intermingled.

I don't believe that the study damaged Upjohn's financial interests. Xanax became one of the most prescribed benzodiazepines. But Upjohn had expected a slam-dunk, not an expensive miss. It's easy to see why they felt disappointed. But results are results, even when you don't like them. That's a bitter pill that researchers and drug makers alike have to swallow time and time again. I saw it happen again to Upjohn in a separate drug trial on social phobia. This time, results were simply accepted.

I take off my hat to the volunteers who made the London-Toronto study possible. They put up with time-consuming procedures while feeling most unwell. They also endured a six-months of follow-up without seeking any additional help. That requires a lot of self-discipline and mountains of goodwill. Which brings me to another issue: They were members of the public. They supported our research, as other members of the public do elsewhere. It stands to reason that research data harvested with the help of the public should be accessible to the public, even when they disappoint.

And, as detective Colombo was fond of saying, there's still "one more thing:" Drug efficacy is usually reported as statistically significant. "Significant" is not the same as "genuinely helpful." Significance is a statistical finding, not proof of substantial health benefits. *"Clinical effectiveness"* describes the latter far better. Clinical effectiveness has been defined as a reduction of symptoms by some 50%. Life does indeed get better at that level of improvement. Drug makers should make the measure available to prescribing physicians.

What else can we learn from this story? I am not against drug trials or the public's participation in them, no matter how critical the above may sound. Quite the contrary: We would be in deep trouble without them. They make prescription drugs safer to use and their benefits more predictable than untested remedies that are backed by little more than a hope and a promise. Volunteers get a crack at an experimental treatment that wouldn't be available otherwise. And I wouldn't miss the Xanax trials for anything. They sharpened my clinical skills, facilitated my own research and improved the accuracy of my medico-legal work.

They also have me throw a hissy fit when politicians recommend a drug because of a vague feeling in their gut.

15.OTHER RESEARCH

Car Accidents And Ptsd

Drug studies like the one just cited are highly organized and tightly controlled. **Exploratory research** is more off the cuff, more like panning a riverbed for gold. Maybe you'll find something, maybe you don't. Our research on car accidents was like that. We didn't know what we would find, only that car accidents deserved a closer look. 1.3 million are reported annually around the world. In the USA, annual economic costs are roughly 242 billion dollars (US Department of Transportation, 2010). That's a lot of cash, a lot of pain, suffering and litigation. Many survivors suffer for years. The first step in our investigation was obvious. When and where and under what circumstances do symptoms occur and how do they impact daily lives? Pain patterns offered no obvious clues, but anxiety and GSR (galvanic skin) response did (see "biofeedback). From a behaviorist's perspective the next step was obvious: Examine the "scene of the crime" like a detective would and go for a ride with a survivor. That did the trick. Anxious survivors startle, duck and shout warnings in traffic situations that wouldn't bother most of us. They sweat and their heart rates shoot up. They are excessively security-conscious and have nightmares of accidents. A sizeable percentage improve with exposure to riding in cars and lessons in safe driving, just like agoraphobics improve with instructions on how to cope with anxiety and walking the streets. A positive response to exposure therapy is characteristic for phobic anxiety. This and characteristic reactions to driving were the reason for naming this symptom cluster **accident phobia**.

My observations began in the mid-seventies and continued for decades. To the best of my knowledge, our first paper (PTSD after motor vehicle accidents, Can. J Psychiatry 1985) was a "first" in the medical literature. Publication wasn't easy. That's unsurprising for something completely novel. Two psychiatric journals rejected our manuscript. A third, the Canadian Journal of Psychiatry, accepted it after a lengthy review. Publication set a process in motion that led to the development of a treatment manual published by the American Psychological Association. Then we dug deeper: Was it wrong to blame our survivors' anxiety on their accident? Had they been anxious before? That's a million-dollar question, as any lawyer will tell you. Subsequent research for the *Accident Fear Questionnaire (AFQ, 1995)* revealed that this wasn't so. Accident phobia was as common in men as it was in women (Statistically, more women than are expected to be phobic within the general population), a finding that suggests a causative link between accident and phobia. The AFQ lists characteristic fears and changes in behavior, harvested from hours of direct observation of traumatized survivors in cars. To validate our findings in reference to PTSD, Brian Cox and myself compared AFQ results with other assessment procedures for PTSD. We found a match. We also found that *behavioral data (changes in driving habits) identified PTSD more reliably than survivors' complaints*. In other words: A change in driving habits tells you more about the presence of PTSD than a general interview will. "Behavior doesn't lie" is a rule of thumb that's proven helpful many times over, as the following chapter will also show.

Meta-Analysis

is another valuable research tool. It pools data from published studies and re-analyzes them. The psychologist Steven Taylor masterminded such a study on PTSD. He re-analyzed data sets from Canadian peacekeepers and survivors of car accidents to identify the "core symptoms" of PTSD that both groups shared, regardless of the large differences in their traumatic experiences. His study identified the PTSD symptoms survivors from *any* traumatic experience have in common. It bolstered the standing of PTSD as a valid psychiatric diagnosis, if used according to validated diagnostic criteria.

Stories about "PTSD" can be outright misleading if the term is used uncritically: "Trauma" means different things to different people, as does "stress" and "disorder." Being the target of unkind words isn't the same order as being in a frightening accident, a war or a concentration camp. "Stress" is more than feeling on edge. It's a bodily reaction along with a psychological one. And "disorder" equals disruption of normal daily functions.

Noisy Data

Psychiatric diagnoses are more than names. They must fulfill clearly defined diagnostic criteria for a listing in the DSM (Diagnostic & Statistical Manual of the American Psychiatric Association). Criteria for a valid diagnosis include a lack scatter (statistical noise). An absence of scatter looks like a single bullet hole hitting the "bull's eye" (read diagnostic criteria) of the target. Wide scatter looks like buckshot fired from afar, with many hits off target. Wide scatter renders a diagnosis dubious, particularly symptoms overlap with the symptoms of another disorder. The more scatter there was, the less a clinician could expect to know about the illness' natural course and treatment. One multicenter study (1987) examined *generalized anxiety disorder* in this regard with the help of several psychometric measures and the aforementioned SCID. The diagnosis survived for the time being, and generalized anxiety disorder remained listed in DSM.

Chronic pain is another "noisy" diagnosis. It's challenging to clinical care and insurers alike. According to NIH (The National Institute for Complementary and Integrative Health), close to 20% of US adults complain of chronic pain at some point in their lives, and some 8% complain of "high-impact pain," the kind that kept the Smythe Pain Clinic busy. This and the Ontario Government's concern over injured workers' compensation inspired a *systematic review of the entire scientific literature* on chronic pain to answer the following questions: *How valid is it as a clinical diagnosis? How credible is it for purposes of compensation? And how efficacious are currently available methods of diagnosis and treatment?* The "systematic" aspect of the study indicated a lack of "cherry picking" and "confirmation bias," achieved by including all published studies from the world literature. It included only peer-reviewed publications and studies that followed their subjects prospectively (going forward). The Government of Ontario, the Ministry of Health and Welfare and the Workers Safety and Insurance Board of Ontario sponsored the project.

It was a tall order. A team of librarians assembled thousands of publications. A second team of statisticians reviewed data quality. A third team of experienced researchers and clinicians reviewed the studies that had passed muster, then conferenced them to reach a consensus. It was an unparalleled enterprise that included a neurosurgeon, an orthopedic surgeon, a physiatrist, a physiotherapist, an occupational therapist, a chiropractor and myself as the lone shrink. The Clinical Journal of Pain published the resulting monograph in 2001. The monograph reaffirmed chronic pain as a valid health issue and summarized promising interventions. The study may have influenced Ontario's workers' compensation policies, hereby confirming the need for an evidence-based review before health care policy is made.

16. SWEATING
IT IN COURT

The Courts of Law represent the supreme power of the State. Lives change when the gavel comes down. Some verdicts also set "precedent." They influence future cases for years to come, as Jane Roe did vs. Henry Wade. Witnesses must show up when summoned (subpoenaed), or they face a charge of contempt punishable by jail. Jurors must be independent, impartial and take direction only from the judge. Doctors under summons must produce their medical records and whatever else that's considered relevant to the case. If attendance disrupts their schedule and upsets their patients, if they have to work longer hours and burn the midnight oil to make up for time lost, that's their problem. Once on the stand, they swear (or affirm) that they will say "nothing but the truth and only the truth," mindful of the fact that lying under oath is a criminal offense. They must answer a multitude of difficult questions and face a cross-examiner who will do her best to tear their expertise apart, leaving their egos a smoldering ruin. In Ontario, the Scales of Justice, the Lion, the Unicorn and the Crown remind you of this. It's small wonder then that doctors duck out of sight at the first hint of having to testify. And duck I did for years, until a murder case changed my mind. A Crown attorney was prosecuting an (alleged) murderer whose paper-thin defense defied scientific reasoning. Refusing him assistance felt like a cop-out. If I have a creed, it's that scientific reasoning should prevail. I shifted from ducking to being scrupulously prepared. If I had to go to Court, it was to feed the lions, not to be fed to them.

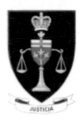

Ontario Court General Division

An "expert witness" is a small cog on the wheels of justice. He doesn't know the Law and doesn't argue it. He only describes what he knows and how he came to know it during his examination-in-chief. If that's all he does, if he simply describes, his cross-examiner may limit herself to a few probing questions. If he goes out on a limb to support one party to the litigation over the other, he may feel like a trembling goat circled by a hungry tigress. Does he possess the relevant qualifications? Is he familiar with the facts of the case? How did he arrive at his opinion? Did a plaintiff's illness really develop as result of the alleged cause? Might she have fallen ill anyway? Why was her illness disabling? What's her prognosis? In a typical case the doctor writes a report to his retaining attorney that covers all this. It will be served to the opposing attorney before the trial, who then has his own expert go over it in reply. In contentious cases a battle may ensue between opposing experts, with reports going back and forth until the matter is either settled out of court or by trial.

Forensic interviewing is not a relaxed affair. Plaintiffs were understandably reluctant when I interviewed them on behalf of the Defense. Defendants were cautious, but never aggressive when I examined them on behalf of the Crown. My style was "soft," similar to what's been called "befriending" by detectives. To me, this made a lot of sense. It gets people to talk. And it's important to look at both sides of the story, important also to let the interviewee know that. Once it helped me out of a situation that could have been dangerous. I was interviewing a defendant in a maximum-security facility on behalf of the Crown when an administrative snafu occurred. There I was, in a small open-door office, surrounded by an open area with restless prisoners pacing back and forth, without security personnel anywhere in sight. A small riot and general lockdown had occurred the day before and a feeling of unease still lingered. Around us wandered various inmates looking tetchy. A few looked in on the two of us, with us waving friendly hands at them. We were getting on well according to all appearances, and that may have saved me from being taken hostage, or whatever else somebody bigger than I may have had in mind. I came away from the experience a little wiser. Being locked up behind several layers of steel doors and bars with next to no contact with the outside world must be maddening. Considering the gravity of these circumstances, balance and objectivity are as vital to the accused as they are to the victim.

The hallways in Toronto's Superior Court are busy places. Junior lawyers in long black gowns cart stacks of documentation. Senior counsels gather in small groups and whisper confidences. Judges won't be seen until they appear in full regalia to calls of "all rise," which we dutifully do. For me the routine rarely varied. A retaining letter on top of a stack of files would arrive in banker's boxes months before the trial. It might hold a thousand pages or more, some in barely legible handwriting, also pictures and sometimes evidence from surveillance. I would look through these before examining the plaintiff (or defendant). He might be friendly and cooperative or distant and adversarial, depending on his mood and the circumstances of the case.

I would ask him to complete a set of psychometrics prior to the interview and complete a second set myself based on direct observation. I'd ask diagnostic questions as determined by the Diagnostic Manual (DSM) and get the plaintiff's views on the case. After the interview, I would go over the file a second time with a fine-tooth comb, compare my interview data with data from other sources, look for contradictions, develop a theory of the case and write it all up, papers spread out over tables, chairs and the floor. I would rehearse my testimony the night before the hearing and sleep a broken sleep. Getting to Court on time always was a worry. I always departed early, in anticipation of traffic jams and snowfalls.

Once in Court I would read parts of my report of the page and re-cite the rest from memory. Humor was the judge's exclusive do-main. After the examination-in-chief the dreaded cross-examin-ation would follow. It had me on my toes every time, ready for curveballs. I did my best to anticipate the route a cross-examiner might take and took my time with difficult questions. Anyone who doubts that anxiety has physical consequences should visit the public washroom of a courthouse. The evidence is there to see. And anyone who fears public speaking is in for a special treat.

Most of my cases were "*civil.*" A plaintiff might sue a defendant (by extension his insurer) for monetary damages after a car or industrial accident, or he might sue over (alleged) medical mal-practice. My role (but not my testimony) depended on who had retained me, Plaintiff or Defendant. In the least complicated cases, the plaintiff would be a patient of mine and I would be act-ing for Plaintiff. I would copy of the relevant parts of her medical record to her attorney after receiving a signed release and add a covering letter that summarized her illness, its likely causes, treatment and related disability. I would only write an opinion if it was in her favor. If the Defense retained me, my procedure would be similar. I'd review the relevant medical records and examine the plaintiff with her consent. There I would always write a report. A *summons* (subpoena) by the "opposition" was rare in civil cases. If issued at all, it would be considerate of my time and circumstances. A hostile one was highly unusual.

One summons in a civil case was patently uncivil. It landed on my desk in the middle of winter. I was starved for sun and had a pre-paid vacation to the Caribbean. My pleas for accommodation fell on deaf ears. I had to attend on the stated day, or I would be "in contempt." I tried to negotiate, declared my willingness to attend Court at any time other than the one specified, as this would nix my holiday without a refund. When that failed, I contacted the Law Society of Upper Canada. Counsel from the Law Society had a chat with the issuer of the summons, again to no avail. He wouldn't budge (as was his legal right). Gnashing my teeth, I took a closer look at the hated piece of paper and, eureka, a clerical error had come to my rescue. The summons listed the time of the Court hearing, but not the place. It looked invalid. I checked with a friend in the legal fraternity and left for the Caribbean, snail-mailing a letter to summoning counsel to indicate where I could be reached. I never heard from him again. Another summons was outright punitive. It demanded my personal tax records, going back years. It's fair enough to ask questions about Court-related earnings in cross-examination, to flush out "hacks" that write made-to-order reports for one side only, Plaintiff or Defense. This particular summons demanded records unrelated to any court work. It breached my privacy rights and I wasn't going to have it. Retaining counsel suggested that I bring my personal records to court, sealed and ready for inspection, then ask the judge for a ruling. - The trial concluded without this distraction.

An outright attempt of intimidation occurred only once, during cross-examination. A mother was suing for compensation after her son's fatal road accident. Her demand exceeded the usual provisions of Family Law, and I was retained to testify for the Defense. The media were covering the case and the large court-room was packed. The plaintiff was visibly angry and noisily interrupted proceedings. Counsel for Plaintiff took his cue from her. He approached the witness box where I stood, the villain who dared to imperil his client's claim. His act was flawless. His black gown and long black mane flowed with each step as he approached the witness stand, head held high and dark eyes piercing. Moving ever closer, he fired question after question, shouting the last one in my face from just feet away. He had a reputation for theatrics and he was confirming it. I had parsed my responses up to then. This crossed a line. It was my turn now for theatrics. I paused for effect, then asked him quietly if he "could please speak up a little," this just loud enough for the judge to hear. His Honor smiled ever so slightly, which I took for encouragement. My cross-examiner was not amused. He held aloft his large file and shook it violently, demanding loudly if I knew what "this" was all about. My response was flippant enough to invite censure from his Honor: "Can I wait for the movie?" I asked as quietly as before. His Honor asked me to repeat this out loud, and the courtroom collapsed in laughter. The cross-examination ended shortly afterwards.

Such moments were rare. It's far easier to be the proverbial deer in the headlights. When an Alabama psychiatrist was charged with defrauding Medicare, his defense attorney retained me to challenge the Prosecution's evidence. Its witnesses were former patients. FBI agents had asked them to recall all visits the doctor had billed for. They recalled some, but not all, seemingly confirming the Prosecution's charge of excess billing. I questioned the reliability of their recall. The witnesses had been admitted to a psychiatric ward during the relevant times. They were on tranquillizers known to impair memory. I cited corroborative opinion from a contemporary American textbook, considering that proof enough. The cross-examining State Attorney seemed to go easy on me at first. On closing, he asked innocently if I was a "friend of the defendant." I said so and naively left it at that. The judge then disallowed my testimony as "biased" and my friend was convicted.

The ruling bothered me for years. I should have pushed back with something like "two plus two makes four, even if a friend of the accused says so." I had to learn the ropes, and badly. Experience helped some. Then a legal journal advertised a course on cross-examination at Osgood Law School in Toronto. Nobody asked any questions when I registered there together with a colleague. The instructors found us out soon enough, but it didn't matter. Everyone had a good laugh and they let us stay. The course covered various techniques of roping in a hostile witness in cross-examination. Participants practiced in pairs on each other while being videotaped. We critiqued each other afterwards. The course was an eye-opener: A good cross-examiner asks only questions with predictable answers, never open-ended ones that give the witness any wiggle room. She stalks her prey with questions prefaced by "wouldn't you agree that..." and "isn't it possible that...," questions that have only one likely answer. She corners the witness slowly and from several angles, leaving him in the dark about the trap she is about to spring. Committed by his earlier answers, the witness finally has to choose his poison. He can either accept the cross-examiner's premise, or he can debase his earlier statements. His credibility is gone in either case. Our instructors added one proviso: This should be accomplished without ridicule and denigration. - I liked the course so much, I took it twice.

Discussions with retaining counsel also helped my trial preparations. The defense attorney of the Alabama psychiatrist added a bit of good ole' Southern humor. We sat down at his wood-carved desk in his elegant office adjacent to a historical downtown square in Mobile, and I explained my evidence. Counsel considered it too technical. An Alabama jury couldn't understand this. More fitting language was called for, something the jury could grasp. "Doc," he said plainly, "you got to put the hay where the goats can get at it." His trust in the local security was as low as it was in the jury's intellect. After we were done, he reached under the desk, retrieved his colt, holstered it and accompanied me downstairs to the nearest taxi stand.

In preparation to the Ssenjonga trial (see below) the Crown attorney delivered a different piece of advice, this one dead serious. The case was about AIDS, then still an always fatal illness. Ssenjonga stood accused of willfully infecting his intimate partners with the virus. He had kept them in the dark about his own infection, and he hadn't used precautions. Women's rights were at issue here and that raised the emotional temperature of the trial to a fever pitch. The national media headlined daily proceedings and the case was tilting in the defendant's favor. I was in danger of becoming the white knight riding to the damsels' rescue, not a good idea when sober expert testimony is called for. On the day before my testimony the Crown attorney invited me to a London sidewalk café for a get-to-know chat. It was a sunny afternoon and perfect for people-watching. He pointed out some interesting passers-by, assailants, fraudsters and thieves, some who had been convicted and some that had gotten away. Then came the lesson: "The Law doesn't dish out justice according to fairness and morality as the public sees it." It settles cases on the basis of the evidence and according to existing Law." Period. The lesson was clear enough: Describe your evidence, carefully and objectively, no less and no more.

Sometimes though one gives in to feelings, forgets caution and ignores procedure.

I was working on a Defense report in a civil case and I was late. I was also late with an academic paper, and my patient load was at critical levels. I had worked through a night to finish my Defense report in a timely fashion. Now I wanted it off my desk and out the door. And somehow, in my eagerness, I forgot to proofread three wretched pages. They were full of errors as first drafts often are. All errors were about quotes from a file and labeled as quotes, and none affected my conclusions. That didn't help. The plaintiff complained to the College of Physicians and Surgeons of Ontario. He wasn't my patient as he seemed to imply. I corrected my errors and stated this. It took still took weeks and repeated efforts on my part to persuade the College investigator that she was intervening in an ongoing legal case. Crucifixion averted: The complaint was dismissed without record. But the lesson stuck. I haven't sent out a legal report since then without letting at least one day pass since its writing.

I also made it my practice to accept work on behalf of both Defense and Crown in criminal cases, on behalf of Defense and Plaintiff in civil cases. Working for both sides of the aisle keeps you honest. It can also be risqué. A Plaintiff's attorney might remember testimony from another case I had taken on behalf of Plaintiff, and turn my own words against me in a case I had taken on for the Defense. I was either lucky, or my three rules of reporting saved me from cringing on the stand. They are "describe, describe and then describe some more." Describing means saying what you see, when and where you see it, and how you arrived at your conclusions. It's the attorney's job to argue the case, not the medical expert's. I also didn't call anyone a "fake" or a "liar," no matter how unusual their claim might be. A thorough description is good enough. The Court can come to its own conclusion.

It took me a while to get used to court hearings. After declining to testify in the aforementioned murder case, I refused to testify on behalf of a colleague because the prospect made me nervous. I also refused to appear in person in a high-profile criminal case about a wrongful conviction (R. v. Guy-Paul Morin). There the Appeals Court accepted my written report. Then came my appointment to the German Courts to assess Jewish concentration camp survivors. It was politically sensitive but non-adversarial and had me function as a "Friend of the Court." I could be neutral and support neither State nor Plaintiff. The Ontario Workplace Safety and Insurance Board and its Tribunal required a similar neutral stance. Thereafter, growing experience bolstered my confidence. Eventually publications on psychological trauma and pain attracted requests to testify in high-profile cases. The five criminal cases summarized below are in chronological order. They were well within the borders of my bailiwick of anxiety disorders. In three of them the Defense used term *"panic"* in an attempt to absolve their client from criminal charges. In the fourth (the first one below) the defense used anxiety and a history of heart disease to exempt a police officer from testifying. In the fifth the Crown tried to keep evidence of two grisly murders from the media by claiming that publication might damage the mental health of the general public.

My evidence in these **five criminal cases** may look convincing, even compelling on first sight. "Convincing" falls a long way short from proving guilt to judge and jury beyond reasonable doubt.

Guy Paul Morin (Court of Appeal, 1992)
This case was about a miscarriage of justice.

Homicide detective M was a key witness for the Crown in a murder trial. Cigarette butts had been found near the victim's body, but Morin was a non-smoker. Detective M had kept two notebooks on his case, one for "raw notes" and another for the "final version." By the time of trial, his raw notes could not be located. This was troubling, and the defense appealed Morin's conviction. It wanted to re-examine M under oath to explore his evidence in detail.

The Crown resisted this request. Its experts claimed that M was suffering from PTSD and heart disease and that he couldn't testify for health reasons. He had undergone coronary bypass surgery and was on antihypertensive medication. A Wechsler Memory Scale found him "cognitively impaired due to stress." A second psychological test, the MMPI, was "indicative of somatic delusions." Crucially, the Crown claimed that M might die during cross-examination from a heart attack.

The *Defense* cardiologist disagreed with the Crown's conclusions: M's psycho-pharmacological management was "suboptimal" (polite for ill-advised). It needed improving, and then M could testify. I then examined M. He was polite, brief with his statements and matter-of-fact. He did not look anxious during the interview but reported symptoms of hyperventilation and panic anxiety related to an earlier car accident. I couldn't confirm the remainder of the Crown psychologist's report. In my view, M feared heart attacks, which is typical for someone with panic anxiety. It doesn't amount to actual danger from heart attacks. His "anxiolytic" medication of Secobarbital was indeed "suboptimal." - M would be able to testify once his doctor prescribed an appropriate anxiolytic.

The judge ruled that M could testify in an informal setting. This he did and without ill effect. Morin's first appeal however was denied. - A second appeal included DNA evidence. Morin was finally exculpated.

R v Ssenjonga (1993)

This case was about sexual assault by passing on an AIDS infection, by implication also about women's rights in the context of intimate relations. It was a first of its kind in Canada and expected to set precedent.

Ssenjonga had AIDS. His physician informed him of the diagnosis and the local health authority ordered him to refrain from unprotected intercourse. S then (allegedly) infected several women with AIDS. He had not alerted them to his illness before consorting with them. He had also failed to use precautions, this in contravention of the health order.

S was suffering from a rare strain of AIDS. That identified him as the source of his victims' AIDS infection. By the time he was criminally charged, he was suffering from bacterial infections, fevers and a skin condition. He hoped to stay out of jail until he died.

The Crown alleged that S had acted in wanton disregard for his victims' health and safety.

The Defense claimed that S was suffering from PTSD and was therefore unable to "appreciate" the risk of passing his AIDS to others. The origins of his PTSD dated back to the Ugandan War.

He was "traumatized" then by watching Idi Amin's troops beat up civilians. He was "traumatized" again when his doctor told him that he was going to die of AIDS. Psychometrics and neuro-psychological testing "supported" the diagnosis of PTSD. PTSD-related "dissociative phenomena and denial" had rendered S incapable of using proper (sexual) judgment.

Essentially, this was an insanity defense.

The Crown: My examination included the Structured Clinical Interview (SCID), the Impact of Events Scale (which quantifies impairment of daily living) and a behavioral assessment. It did not confirm the Defense diagnosis of PTSD. (I also argued that the Defense psychometrics were not designed to diagnose PTSD.) Admittedly, S had experienced panic anxiety, but only in situations he perceived as confining. He wasn't "phobic" of sexuality and perfectly capable of discussing AIDS-related topics. He lacked social anxiety and was perfectly capable to say "no" to sexual advances. He also did not harbor abnormal fears of violence, which ruled out PTSD after assault. - Illness and the threat of jail explained his current distress, not PTSD.

During my lengthy interview, S described his actions as "immature, like the actions of a little boy." Being criminally charged "made him realize that he had erred." (This confession came close to a guilty plea. It was inadmissible as evidence.) S came across as a sociable man, friendly, vocal and persuasive, this despite the dire straits he was in. I bumped into him again during a break during the trial. He greeted me like an old acquaintance.

During the ensuing trial, _Counsel for the Defense_ cross-examined me for a day-and-a-half in front of a packed courtroom. I few items stand out in memory. Counsel suggested that only psycho-analysts could judge (Freudian) "mechanisms of defense" like dissociation and denial. Consequently I (the non-analyst) wasn't qualified to testify on the matter. I countered by stating that I had read Freud in the German original, whereas his experts had read him in a disputed translation. Counsel (rightly) pointed out that frequent discussion had improved S' ability to talk about

AIDS. I pointed out that evidence of past and present PTSD was lacking. There wasn't much there to "improve," adding that S's actions weren't compelled by psychiatric illness (as in an insanity defense). They were his choice. Counsel then examined my knowledge of PTSD, citing various psychiatric textbooks and journals piled intimidatingly high on a table in front of him. His timing was unlucky. I had published on PTSD shortly before the trial and knew most of the relevant literature by heart.

The judge had written some 130 pages of his ruling when S died "of unknown causes." The ruling remains undisclosed, despite public demands for its release.

The trial was my baptism of fire. My cross- examiner was widely known for his skills and persistence and media attention was unrelenting. The minutest detail mattered. On the second day of testimony the judge had me re-state earlier testimony to calm public furor over a misquote. I sweated it to such an extent the Crown Attorney donated a new shirt to the cause.

The well-known journalist June Callwood' (14) chronicled the matter. Her book "Trial without End" details S' history and the trial fairly, but omits the clash between psychoanalytic theory and clinical psychiatry.

R v Appleton (1994)

In this case, an implied insanity defense relied on theories about "panic" and the unconscious mind.

A stood accused of murdering his mother-in-law in her home. She had sustained five bullet wounds from a homemade, un-rifled and untraceable handgun before hammer blows to the head ended her life. On the night of the murder, A's father-in-law returned late from work. He found his spouse in a pool of blood, called 911 and attempted resuscitation.

A had been invited for dinner that night. He claimed that he was late himself. When he arrived, he saw police at his in-laws' residence and did not enter. Subsequently, homicide detectives retrieved blood evidence from his car and his clothing. They also retrieved a bloodstained dollar bill from a Hasty Market where he had bought fresh clothing shortly after the murder, earning A the nickname of "Hasty Bill." When confronted with the blood evidence, A changed his story: He had found mother-in-law at the scene before the police arrived, tried to revive her and then fled in a "panic," fearing he might be falsely accused of murder. "Panic" also explained his later hiding of blood evidence.

A's family continued to believe in his innocence.

The Crown attorney kept a photo of the blood-splattered murder scene above his desk.

The Defense accepted A's explanation of his actions as "panic" and added explanatory details. A was "traumatized" when dogs attacked him at the age of eight during an altercation. He was "traumatized" again when he witnessed his father's stroke. Thereafter he "denied" the existence of events that "looked wrong" to him and "displaced" them in his mind (a psychoanalytic term for forgetting). He expected blame for all wrongs, no matter how unjustified this might be. His evasiveness might make him appear like a guilty person. Instead, it was caused by panic and fear.

The _Crown_ retained my colleague Peter Collins as expert witness, myself also in support of the investigation. A declined all Crown interviews. We went to see him anyway when he was in a cage-like holding cell in the courthouse. He was a fit-looking muscular man, understandably restless and glum. He refused to even make eye contact.

We challenged the credibility of A's defense as follows: A exhibited none of the (DSM) characteristics of _panic disorder._ He had coped with the sight of blood and injury when working at a hospital. Therefore, a _blood-phobia_ didn't explain his flight from the murder scene. He had no demonstrable history of prior anxiety or mood disorder to portrayed him as "thin-skulled" and vulnerable (as the Defense had suggested). He sounded calm on police surveillance tapes before his arrest, even humorous when describing his crepe-soled shoes as "brothel creepers." He became distressed only after having been charged with murder. - Defense reports had used the term "panic" as laypersons would, not as the DSM defines it.

After A's arrest, more incriminating evidence came to light. He had borrowed a manual on building an unrifled firearm from a London/UK library, evidence courtesy of Scotland Yard. He had deceived his current spouse by not revealing two prior marriages to her. And he had motive: His in-laws were affluent, and A's financial records contained evidence of unsustainable spending. Most importantly, he revealed details about the murder to the defense psychiatrist that only the murderer could have known.

A was convicted and sentenced to life. The murder weapon was never found.

R v Bernardo (1995)

In this case, the Supreme Court of Canada set precedent regarding (the media's) freedom of speech, in the example of videotaped recordings of two grisly murders.

B had committed a series of rapes and murders with the assistance of his partner Karla Homulka. He had videotaped the sadistic humiliation of two teenage victims, including their slow and painful death. Once discovered in his attic, the tapes became crucial evidence. Media coverage was explicit and distressing to the victims' families. They wanted coverage to cease and have B's tapes sealed permanently.

Two detectives were tasked with the review of the tapes. They required counseling afterwards. A legal dispute over media access followed. It led to a separate hearing.

The Crown argued for a complete publication ban, to protect the general public from the psychological harm that publication might cause.

The Media objected. They argued for unhindered access to the evidence. A publication ban would interfere with free speech and the public's "right to know" as guaranteed by the Canadian

Constitution. They retained Dr. Allodi and myself to prepare separate reports on verbatim transcripts from the videos, "snuff-tapes" as the underworld likes to call this sort of thing.

Experts for the Crown asserted that victims' families had no choice but to attend Court. To their mind, a public display of the evidence would repeat the assaults. It would aggravate the psychiatric conditions some family members were experiencing. It might also trigger psychiatric conditions in "Jane Doe" (the general public), as the media had been "grossly insensitive" to date.

Experts for the Media noted that heinous crimes were routinely discussed in open Court. Unhindered reporting could be "cathartic," even "educational" to the public. Reportedly, publicity over a British murder case had this effect. Admittedly, the tapes would be distressing to almost anyone if closely viewed. The police detectives had to do this. They had to pay close attention to every single detail in the tapes and had no choice in the matter. The victims' families and the general public did have a choice. They were free to avert their eyes and cover their ears. They could also stay away completely. The Crown experts were over-reaching. Instead of arguing against freedom of speech and the public's right to know, they should discourage attendance by anyone whose health might be endangered by attending the hearing. Obscenity laws provided the necessary safeguards. They already restricted publication to a reasonable extent.

Justice Lesage allowed the audiotaped portion of the evidence into open Court. He limited the visual material to judge, jury and defendant. Upon appeal, *the Supreme Court of Canada* let his ruling stand.

R v Kelly (Court of Appeal, 1998)
This murder case came up for appeal after a key witness (T) recanted her eyewitness testimony years after the trial. She claimed then that her testimony had been a "false memory." K's subsequent Appeals Court case was therefore based on psychiatric grounds. This made it the first such case in Canada since the Sixties and precedent-setting.

K was an undercover RCMP drug squad officer. In 1984 his wife plunged to her death from a high-rise balcony at Palace Pier in Toronto. Her injuries from the long fall obscured any signs of a struggle. A claimed in his defense that her fall had been an accident. But he had taken out a life insurance policy on her before her death and was a big spender short of money. He also had a checkered past. In spite of all this, murder could not be proven without further evidence.

Ms. Taber was K's ex-girlfriend and a close friend of the victim. She came forward as an eye witness to the murder after a lengthy delay, explaining her hesitation as "trying to block the murder from my mind." Her testimony convicted K, and he went to jail. The spellbinder "The Judas Kiss." (15) describes this part of the story. That wasn't the end of it though.

In 1998 T recanted her testimony. She now claimed that she hadn't witnessed the murder at all. The "truth" dawned on her while she was "panicking" on top of a tower. She realized then that her memory had been "nothing but a dream." She accused the police psychiatrist of "hypnotizing" her during her original deposition, lodging a complaint against him and the two detectives who had also been present during her original deposition.

T had moved abroad by the time K's appeal proceeded on the basis of her recantation. She was unavailable for re-examination. The Crown retained me to review the file.

The Defense argued that T's recantation presented new and credible evidence.

The Crown argued that T's recantation was fictitious.

T did have psychiatric symptoms. She feared heights, had been assaulted twice, once before and once after the murder. She had also been in a car crash and was in psychological treatment. All of this suggested the presence of a psychiatric disorder, but not the existence of a "false memory." That was undocumented, unverifiable and unlikely. T may have delayed her original testimony because she didn't want to talk about the murder. Unease in this context is credible and a delay in her testimony perfectly understandable. It's harder to accept how she could accept her memory as "true" for years and perceive it as "false" years later, as hypnotic suggestion induced somehow by the police psychiatrist. It's also unlikely that her new insight came to her on a high place. A high place might have triggered flashbacks of the murder far more likely than a new insight into a "false memory."

My testimony was unopposed. K's appeal failed.

"Trauma" and the unconscious mind

We can't know the contents of the unpublished judgment in R v Ssenjonga. In the other cases, the Crown countered successfully theories about the role of the unconscious mind in criminal acts. It also demonstrated that neither overwhelming fear (PTSD and phobic avoidance), nor a compulsion (as in obsessive-compulsive disorder), nor a delusion (psychosis) had compelled these acts. It's important to note though that the Crown couldn't really disprove Defense theory about the unconscious mind. It's impossible to prove that something doesn't exist. It's only possible to demonstrate that its existence is unlikely, and that probable alternatives exist.

Similar arguments played a role in the criminal trials of two police officers. Policing is potentially traumatic. Officers come face-to-face with gruesome injuries. They may get assaulted and find themselves looking into the muzzle of a gun. Full-blown PTSD must be considered in such cases. One of the two police cases was about **spousal abuse,** the other about **fraud**. The physical evidence was overwhelming, and neither officer met DSM diagnostic criteria for a PTSD. One pleaded guilty after the Crown medical disputed "last stand" psychological defense. The other case went to trial, outcome unknown. In the rape case against the former premier *Gerald Regan* in 2002 before the Supreme Court of Nova Scotia, the psychiatric expert for the Crown advanced once more theories about forgetting and remembering and the unconscious mind of alleged victims. The trial was held *in camera* and I cannot comment further, except that Regan was found not guilty. Let it be said however that eloquently phrased psychoanalytic theory about trauma and the unconscious mind may well impact future cases. Instead of offering more of the same arguments, I made up **a lay cross-examination** to illustrate my point.

A "cat" cross-examines an expert "mouse." The mouse is claiming "trauma and repression" in defense of its client's actions. As you might guess, the cat is a heavy favorite.

"**Cat**: *If I understand you correctly, you are telling the Court that your client suffered a traumatic event years ago, which he repressed. Repressed trauma explains the emotional turmoil he has suffered in recent years and his alleged actions.* **Expert**: *Yes, that's correct.* **Cat**: *Please help me understand the process of repression. Does this happen a lot?* **Mouse**: *I believe so. Repression is common in everyday life. Many people can't recall bad memories but continue to act on them.* **Cat**: *You are very experienced in these matters. Have you seen this happen? Could you describe to me what it looks like when someone is repressing a bad memory?* **Mouse**: *Sorry, I can't. Repression is not something you can see or hear.* **Cat**: *But you are saying that it happens a lot. Have you seen it demonstrated in some way or other, maybe by a laboratory or radiographic test?* **Mouse**: *No, I haven't. I explore repressed memories through careful enquiry.* **Cat**: *Can you demonstrate to the Court how you determine that a client of yours has repressed a memory?* **Mouse**: *I can't. I would have to spend considerable time with the client to do that. There isn't enough time to do this in Court.* **Cat**: *Exactly what would convince you that repression had happened, apart from spending a lot of time?* **Mouse**: *It would be a memory that was lost and is now re-surfacing.* **Cat**: *Can you see or hear this as it happens? What are the signs? How do you make sure the "memory" isn't a phantasy?* **Mouse**: *It's a conclusion I draw on the basis of extensive experience.* **Cat**: *We have gone full circle. You have drawn a conclusion, but on what basis? Please explain why the Court should accept as evidence something that even you, the expert can't see, hear or demonstrate in any reliable way to a third party.* **Mouse** *(before leaving the stand): You should give* *me some credit for my experience.* (The last sentence is a verbatim quote from an actual cross-examination.)

According to the philosopher Karl Popper, a hypothesis (a claim in a legal lingo) is useless unless it can be verified independently. That's a core principle of scientific thinking. The **null hypothesis** embodies it in drug trials and other quantitative research. To my mind, a similar rule should also apply to medical testimony. Testimony should be based on observable facts and these must be open to challenge. Here's my olive branch those who consider my reasoning biased: Should it become possible to observe the process of repression and denial by any means, radiographic, electroencephalographic or otherwise, I will accept it. I have been wrong before. I was wrong in regards to certain kinds of minimal brain injury. That was invisible years ago, and modern radiographic methods have made it visible. Maybe the same will happen with repression, although I doubt it. Until then, repressed trauma and the unconscious mind are as invisible as ghosts are in a haunted house.

During the pre-trial of another murder case, the same issue recurred in a different guise. Counsel cross-examined me about my expert qualifications. His client had claimed **"conversion blindness"** (blindness for psychological reasons) in an earlier matter. He had also been observed picking out his beer bottle from a cluster of others on a crowded pub table. To me, this damaged his credibility. Counsel's initial questions about my practice were routine. Then came the stinger: Had I ever assessed a case of "conversion blindness?" I hadn't and said so, failing to add "credible." I "had no experience in the matter," was counsel's conclusion. My inexperience with conversion blindness "disqualified" me from testifying. Feeling annoyed, I asked if I could "tell him a little story." Counsel agreed, and I replied with a ruse of my own: "When an old farmer went to Court to testify, a lawyer asked him if he had ever seen any flying cows. Being honest, the farmer admits that has never in seen such a thing, not in his entire life. According to counsel's logic, a farmer who has never seen any flying cows is no expert on cows." Counsel gave me a very dirty look and His Honor qualified me.

The Vancouver psychologist and fellow author Steven Taylor summed up of what I have to say on this: It's *cognitive science fiction.*"

Fictitious illness is patently improbable from a diagnostic perspective. It is rare in clinical practice and found mostly in courtrooms. Here are a few: One couple claimed "PTSD" from a collapsing bed, a putative "trauma" without any demonstrable danger or injury. Minor accidents "caused" persistent muteness in three plaintiffs that failed to display any signs neurological abnormality beyond the convenient inability to answer probing questions. One was unmasked by a sting operation, I won't say how. Another plaintiff limped on crutches into my office and walked out later, jumping with joy, this when feeling unobserved. His claim was settled out of court, a cheaper resolution than a successful defense, costly though in terms of the moral hazard this entailed. The following claim over a broken leg was as just fictitious as the others, but more intriguing. The plaintiff's broken leg was straightforward enough, but not the story that went with it. The door to a high-rise garbage depository had been faulty. The plaintiff hadn't noticed this. She locked herself in by accident when she dumped her garbage. When she realized that she was locked in, she felt "claustrophobic." She then climbed into the narrow garbage chute, intending to slide down one floor to exit from there. She then lost her footing, careened all the way down the chute to the ground floor and into a garbage container. She was very lucky. The compactor was turned off and garbage cushioned her fall. The fall broke her leg, and her claim of "claustrophobia" broke her credibility: No genuine claustrophobic would escape from one small space by squeezing herself into a much smaller one, at least none I have ever seen.

Nothing ever made my day like "Subway Elvis" did, a busker who performed years ago in Toronto subway stations. Elvis wasn't faking. He was the unlucky suspect in an armed bank robbery near Toronto. A masked man in an Elvis costume had committed it. Subway Elvis was charged with the crime, convicted and did time, this on shaky evidence as it turned out. An alibi exonerated him and the Crown Law Office found itself in the unhappy role of defending HRM and the Canadian taxpayer against a claim for wrongful conviction. When Elvis came to see me for the mandatory medical, I expected the usual disgruntled plaintiff who didn't want to be there. How wrong I was. "Elvis is here!" was the receptionist's breathless announcement. And there he was in full regalia, black hair slicked back and gleaming, with over-sized dark-rimmed sunglasses, in a white imitation leather jacket festooned with bells that jingled with every movement, bellbottom pants and two-tone shoes. He carried a guitar and offered to perform. I loved his gumption. Sadly, I had to carry out my boring duties and never got to hear his proffered "love me tender, love me sweet…" And I did have to "let him go."

My next medico-legal was already pacing in the waiting room.

17.THE RUBBER CHICKEN CIRCUIT

Suppose you have done some research and have a bit of a messianic bend, wouldn't you want to shout it from the rooftops? Standing at a podium in Montreal's big arena was my big chance. The arena can hold a crowd of three thousand. Looking down from the dizzying height of the lectern, I could believe it. The place was buzzing. People were chatting, moving seats, walking in and out. I was going to say a few introductory words at a public forum on anxiety and felt like a clinical example of it. I didn't get a rock star's reception either. Two or three stock French sentences didn't turn any heads. I switched to English, hoping to do better with a story about a long-departed aunt, proverbial in the family for her terror of being late for trains. My disconnect with the crowd continued. Another speaker took over after my allotted five minutes. He got a similar reception. The audience finally came to life during the question-and-answer part of the forum. Then questions came thick and fast. It almost felt like fun. After it was all over, our corporate sponsors rewarded us with a non-Clintonesque sum.

After the launch of the Anxiety Disorders Clinic, requests to participate in forums, shows and roundtables trickled in. Most were phone-ins on the radio. It was hard to connect with an unseen audience, harder still to do this from home while holding a cup of tea. TV studios were easier. I could make eye contact with the host and get feedback. Coaches tell you to sound confident on these occasions but not grand, and to avoid hard-to-pronounce words that might trip you up. They suggest looking straight into the lens, make love to the camera and avoid sideways glances. These might look shifty. I tried to imagine the caller's face and talk to her as if chatting with an old friend. There wasn't much conversation though. Phone-ins allowed one reply per caller before moving to the next one in the line-up. Humor could be toxic and gossip was ill advised. I was more than cautious. I was wooden. When the moderator wasn't with me in the studio I felt isolated. On one occasion I was all-alone in a cubbyhole in one of the CBC's old buildings in downtown Toronto. Cardboard boxes lined the wall behind me. A camera pointed at my face. The moderator was a thousand miles away in Alberta. A light came on when we went live. Presumably a picture of Toronto was inserted behind my head. A background of cardboard boxes would have been more realistic. Afterwards I was told that millions watched the show (probably while eating lunch).

Publicity can be a great ego trip. Colleagues tell you with newly found respect that they saw you on TV. Strangers say hello on the subway. TV stations fetch you in a stretch limousine. You meet famous people. Leonard Nimoy of "Star Trek" fame wanted to rent my office for a movie with a psychiatric theme. Was someone pulling my leg? I agreed on the spot when his assistant called. The story of "The Good Mother" was set in New England. Toronto was the production site. Mr. Nimoy was directing and Dianne Keaton played the lead. Gargantuan trucks pulled up on the appointed day for the stars to spend their downtime in. I met the famous one and noted a lack of pointy ears. Then movers put my antique furniture into storage and replaced them with a version of "early Holiday Inn" (an old insult to Henry Kissinger's taste in furnishings). The lime lights came on and the actors emerged from their mobile living rooms." The villain of the plot was a psychiatrist. He was cold and devoid of empathy, not the kind I would like to represent my profession. I had facilitated my own symbolic hanging. But watching a movie in the making was exiting. And it paid more than my practice would during the time it took to shoot the psychiatric scenes.

After the dust-up in Geneva, Upjohn cold-shouldered me. Another drug company, Myers Briggs, took up the slack. They invited me to a visit at their research facility in Wallingford, New Jersey, a couple of hours drive from New York. The night before, visitors were lodged in a very nice hotel at the United Nations Plaza where watching aloof diplomats is a pastime. Myers-Briggs were researching "*lazarones*" in Wallingford, a novel class of agents so named because they might resurrect dying tissue after strokes and heart attacks (sorry, no further news). Hamster forebrains were isolated from their blood supply to model impending cell death. The research was closely held and staff were not allowed to take any written or electronic information outside the building. They hadn't lost their sense of humor though and put on a dazzling show of "pharmaco-theatre." It included the memorable claim that the brain contains more synapses than the galaxy has stars, each synapse secreting at least five different neurotransmitters. The audience was suitably impressed.

Myers Briggs made *Buspirone*, a non-sedating tranquillizer, potentially useful to anxious people who must remain both calm and on high alert. Nervous drivers, anxious operators of machinery and edgy soldiers might benefit from it. It might save the lives of freshly trained combat troops that would otherwise "freeze" in terror when faced with a mortal threat. The idea interested the US Army and exited newscasters. Sometime after my visit to Wallingford, a US Army officer turned up at Anxiety Disorders to pick Richard's and my brains on the matter. He was discreetly dressed in civvies, but might as well have turned up in full uniform with an ID tag. His crew cut, the razor-sharp crease in his trousers and boots polished to a mirror shine were a dead give-away. I liked his laid-back posture, alert mind and medical authorship reminiscent of my old supervisor in Gainesville.

Nothing came of the visit. It might have been too hot to handle anyway.

This was the big time, if you want to call it that. The rest of the circuit was decidedly down-market. I volunteered for live talks to the general public in libraries and classrooms. Few people trickled in. Most of them sat as far from the speaker as possible. The coffee was basic drip, the cookies hard. An early partner in these ventures was a Toronto psychologist named Quirk. Introduced to audiences as "Kook & Quirk," we extolled on the merits of behavior therapy and systematic desensitization. I also joined Ray Evans from the Pain Clinic for pain rounds with doctors and nurses sponsored by the Ministry of Health. They were held in remote communities and included interviews with live patients. Sometimes it seemed the local doctors had beaten the bushes for the most vexing cases, guaranteed to stump the bigwigs from Toronto.

After Upjohn's requests for talks on *Xanax* dried up. Talks on behalf of Myers Briggs on *Buspirone* took their place. The routine was always the same. I would get a call about an upcoming event. A rep would pick me up at the appointed time and drive me north to a small community somewhere in the rocky landscape of the Canadian Shield. There a handful of doctors would attend my dog-and-pony show on *Buspirone* and behavioral medicine, the latter part of the program on my insistence. A promise of supper and a bit of socializing encouraged attendance. Occasionally we hopped on a short-haul flight. I saw places far away from tourist routes, places I would have never visited otherwise. Unforgettable was a drive in the northern prairies under a fall sky shortly after the harvest during an incredibly long sunset. Bales of straw stood out like torches against darkening fields. A doc took me to a fur traders' warehouse in Northern Ontario. It was filled with rich pelts from wolves, bears, caribou and beaver, covering rows and rows of tables and shelves. They represented an important source of income to the native community, to be sold by auction during the following days. Other docs had tall stories to tell. "How many cars does it take on a cold winter day to fog in an intersection in South Porcupine? - Only two." "How does one land a small plane on a snow-white frozen lake that blends into a white horizon? - Very, very gently, while praying that the altimeter is working just fine." (It didn't in one case, and Innuit snowmobilers came to the rescue.) "What's the most common traffic accident in Ontario's North? - Moose against snowmobile." (A bedded down moose meets a snow-mobile head-on as it rounds a bend.) There was a lot to admire about medical practice in remote communities, dedication, grit and managing with small resources. Some northern family doctors look after many hundreds of patients, with few specialists to back them up. When one of them wants to take time off, the others must cover her clinic visits, night calls and emergencies. That's hard when numbers are small. Single docs are also not allowed to date their patients, past or present, or the College will come down on them like a ton of bricks. That leaves singles with few options. In the resigned words of one: "I might as well thumb it on the highway."

Supper and an opportunity to socialize were an integral part of most corporate-sponsored events, with deep-fried chicken on the menu or local fare. I became expert on "chicken fingers" (if there's such a thing) and anything melted onto toast. Usually, we had a full house. Once though an entire audience cancelled at short notice. The planned presentation was a multi-disciplinary review of stress and the heart. Three university-based specialists, had flown in, a cardiologist, an internist and myself. Drug advertisement was limited to a small display on a side table. The arrangement was as academically pure as driven snow. The sponsor was not amused by the sudden cancellation. Rumor had it that local politics plus a lack of food and drink were to blame. The three of us went ahead anyway and lectured each other. It was one of the best courses I ever attended and my smallest audience ever, also the most responsive. Only one presentation had been as poorly attended before, this one at a high-powered academic conference in Ottawa. A group of behaviorists were offering an update on treatment techniques, and only four or five psychiatrists attended. The rest of our audience had gone AWOL, to pack a conference room next door on sex therapy.

Drug advertisement by doctors is *verboten* nowadays by Ontario's College rules. I don't regret my time on the circuit though, given the variety and down-to-earth discussions with family doctors it provided.

18.WHO'S NEXT?

Decades ago, I visited Sigmund Freud's office at the Berggasse in Vienna. Shelves crammed with books, pictures, masks, antiques and soft light filtered by heavy curtains gave it an aura of mystery and thoughtful exploration. Something groundbreaking had happened there. For the first time in modern psychiatric history could patients claim the undivided attention of a doctor for hours at a time. Freud's observations and those of his followers deepened our understanding of Western culture. His theory guided the practice of psychotherapy for decades to come. I couldn't help acquiring a nostalgic attachment to the scene.

My Viennese cabbie didn't agree. To him, Freud's work was gibberish.

Other psychiatrists have doubled as philosophers, Karl Jaspers on existentialism, Carl Jung on symbolism and the collective unconscious, neo-Freudians like Alfred Adler, Eric Fromm and Karen Horney on society and culture. Their proclivity towards insight and reflection seemed worth perpetuating. Unfortunately, the ambience of Anxiety Disorders, the mood disorders clinic at the Royal Victoria Hospital in Barrie and the Smythe Pain Clinic at TGH was a very far cry from Freud's *Berggasse*. And modern psychiatrists are just as short of time as other medical specialists. Our clinics were like any medical practice, devoted to symptom relief and rehabilitation, not introspection.

They used computers and databases instead of pen and paper, contained steel-and-plastic hospital-issue furniture and examination tables, not armchairs, couches, paintings, handmade carpets and African masks. The Smythe Pain Clinic didn't smell of pipe. It smelled of antiseptics, was part of the Department of Anesthesia and located next door to a surgery ward. All three clinics were booked solid months in advance and their schedules planned to the minute. You couldn't get any further away from analytic couches and the unconscious mind. I hankered for years for the comforts of a refuge removed from rigid schedules, crises and the incursions of hospital administrators. It materialized finally on the ground floor of a crumbly Victorian building in downtown Toronto. Clients came there for CBT (cognitive-behavioral therapy) and behavior therapy, but also just to talk.

The home office was on the ground floor, its entrance next to a back alley and identified by nothing more than a small nametag. That made it attractive to anyone who didn't want to be seen dead in a psychiatric facility. It had two large stained-glass windows, two fireplaces, Art Deco plaster, antique furniture and a few sculptures, a throwback to Siegmund's romantic old days. I didn't have a receptionist and made all appointments in person. The door to the waiting room was unlocked to the street and clients let themselves in. The arrangement had its risks, tolerably so as it turned out. Only three people walked in unannounced over some twenty years. One sat on my doorstep early one morning, just as I was leaving for the hospital. He was severely distressed and I was glad he had come. The other two were of a different kind. One made clinking noises in the waiting room. I found a lad there in his twenties, a trainee burglar who pretended to be a workman. He was nervous and almost apologetic when I asked to look into his tool bag. He muttered something and left. The second intruder was a pro. He was bulky, scowled menacingly and had a prison pallor. He snuck through the waiting room into the private part of the house and upstairs to my apartment. He smashed a lock there to get in, but failed. His efforts made enough noise to have me running upstairs. I approached him with caution and stepped aside as he hurried back downstairs, out the front door and into a waiting get-away car.

Apart from these two interludes, peace reigned. Some very accomplished people asked for my advice within these walls. I sometimes felt like an imposter, regardless of the degrees and certificates on my wall. I learned more from clients on some days than they learned from me. I saw predominantly Anglos, also people from North Africa and Asia. Women outnumbered men, probably because phobias – a major part of my practice - affect women more commonly than men. I saw many university-educated clients, probably because they were more accepting of behavior therapy than others. I may not have had much diversity, but I had variety. My practice included ladies of the night who enlightened me on the meaning of a "golden shower" and pulled hourly wages that exceeded mine by an enviable margin. At the hospital, it included an anti-psychiatry provocateur who tried to trick me into signing a form for involuntary hospital admission by faking delusions. It included a curry-eating plaintiff who tried to fend off unwelcome questions and a nervous mobster with a security detail. He had been shot up badly, and his bodyguard was packing heat. A self-declared "hit man" also wanted help with occupational stress. His jacket didn't bulge under his armpit, and that enabled a very polite conversation.

Most clients combined depression and anxiety with physical symptoms like gastro-intestinal discomfort, faintness, dizziness, breathlessness or palpitations, usually aggravated by a crisis. Just listening seemed to help. Whenever fitting and in opposition to the "medical" approach, I borrowed from *Gestalt therapy* (4): A client had to "own" her problem. She had to take responsibility for it, instead of blaming it on irremediable illness and circumstance. Once she had shifted from expressions of helplessness and was preparing to take charge, collaborative intervention became possible. What were her most troubling symptoms? How did these impact her life? Were there any important any activities she could no longer pursue? Which ones needed restoring? How should this be done? I functioned like a plumber consulting with a home owner on a leak. I discussed options, strategy, self-help techniques based on behavioral principles and prescribed drugs whenever symptoms were incapacitating. With phobics, a short "course" on coping with severe anxiety would follow, then instructions for graded self-exposure. In social phobia, social context and cognitive therapy played a more prominent role.

Method is as important in psychotherapy as it is in research. It keeps you on track. Imagine yourself in the middle of nowhere, very much on your own and a bit confused, without a clear idea of where to go from there. That's how many people feel in the beginning. It's good then to be handed a compass that points towards a goal. Once the goal was defined, markers and milestones were added to tell the client how she was progressing on her way there. Mood and feelings are important during this journey. They can't be the main guide. A client might otherwise change medications or therapists on a lousy day, then wonder later why she did it. Objective markers provide better feedback. How many hours of good sleep is she getting? What's happening with her most important activities? Descriptive feedback that uses behavioral observations is less "noisy" than short-lived emotion, particularly if observations are monitored as *averages* per week. It can take weeks for antidepressant effects to kick in, far longer still for psychotherapy. It's important to play the long game and not give in to impulsive decision-making, or you'll be going in circles.

Interpersonal conflict is a common source of apprehension, and apprehension creates more heat than light. A bit of introductory theorizing encourages a more detached mindset. Exactly what problem needs solving? What would success look like? What will it take to get there? Suppose an employee wants a raise at work, while fearful of antagonizing her boss. Technically speaking, hers is an *approach/avoidance conflict*. She badly wants a raise. She also dreads confrontation. How then will she approach this touchy subject? Good reconnaissance is essential before trying anything. How much money do others make in similar positions? Does her employer appreciate her work performance? How can she tell? How replaceable would she be? How much understanding can she expect from senior management if she bargains? What kind of a settlement would be realistic? How should she phrase her request? Rehearsal and role-play can be useful there: How does her request sound to her when she voices it out loud? Is it too timid or too brusque? How would she feel if she were on the receiving end? In a second scenario, she might be offered a transfer she'd rather not accept but should, if she wants to stay good terms with her boss. Technically speaking, that's an *avoidance/avoidance conflict*. She doesn't want the transfer and she doesn't want to upset her boss. Again, reconnaissance comes first. Is this an offer she can't refuse? What would resigning do to her career? Should she ask for something in return, something like a raise? Should she ask for a more suitable transfer? How have others fared in similar situations? A third scenario represents a nicer kind of conflict, an *approach/approach conflict*: You like both choices but can have only one. Indecision is the main problem there. Flipping a coin may be better than prevaricating endlessly. Socrates took a sardonic view on this in the case of an indecisive young man that contemplated marriage. "Do what you like. You'll regret both."

Guided imagery can assist rehearsal with all kinds of decisions. You lie back and "run a movie" of the task or scene in question. Pair it with relaxed breathing as you run the movie in your mind. Vary it until you like its looks. A therapist can help with the imagery. She can't do it for you. I took a course in hypnotherapy once, hoping for a more powerful technique, but was unconvinced. The course added persuasion and mystery to the procedure, but nothing useful.

Behavioral concepts may sound touchingly simple. "My secretary could do this," said one departmental head dismissively.

To me, this was praise: Psychotherapy must be mystery-free and user-friendly. I recommended Isaac Marks' " Living with Fear" (16, see also 17) for self-help with phobias, Claire Weekes' books (9) on self-help with anxiety and the "One Minute Manager" series by Ken Blanchard and Spencer Johnson for help with daily action plans. Pavlov's dogs illustrated how **classical conditioning** (pairing two stimuli, food with the sound of a bell) produces involuntary reactions like salivation, nausea or dizziness. With PTSD, similar conditioning may take place: Assault elicits terror. Both become linked, and reminders of the assault trigger terror thereafter. If a client feels that classical conditioning makes sense in her circumstances, behavioral intervention is self-explanatory (de-conditioning by desensitization). Therapy then resembles an open-label drug trial. You test the proposed treatment along predefined outcome criteria (declining anxiety responses to reminders of assault), to see if it works. And if it doesn't, you look for a better theory.

Occasionally, an experience tells you more than a thousand words. I chose a reflex that requires no prior conditioning to explain **placebo** responses to a group of eager medical students: The Dollar Store used to sell a gooey substance called "Slime." It looked like snot or worse, perfect for the demonstration of a reflexive gut response. I poured its fanciest version, greenish bits of gob with pink worms amongst them, into a hospital-issue kidney dish, making it look like it came from a ward, then told them to watch me closely. I stuck a finger in it, licked it and asked them how they felt. A few felt nauseous and slightly faint, without having tasted or touched the stuff themselves. They were living examples of the reflexive responses suggestion can elicit.

Questions about quality of life can be explored by another behavioral concept, B.F. Skinner's *operant conditioning through reinforcement,* aka *rewards, nudges* and *incentives* (18). "**Know your reinforcers**" is Skinner's motto. Positive reinforcers (pleasure) fuel motivation. Money is a prime example. It's an almost universal reinforcer that can buy many other reinforcers. Most ordinary mortals are prepared to work for it, provided the amount is right. Several books describe its role in more detail from an economist's perspective, including Steven Levitt and Stephen Dubner's "Think Like A Freak" (19) and Tim Harford's "The Undercover Economist" (20). Billionaires probably won't work for money, at least not for the amounts motivate the rest of us. They have lots of the stuff already. Billionaires might work for attention though. It's probably the most universal reinforcer of them all. Advertisers base their business on it. Demonstrators may raise hell for the sake of it. Facebook and Twitter would be dead in the water without it. Even your dog wants it. Conversely, a lack of attention is political death, withholding it one of the most potent punishments. Ask yourself what your reinforcers are and how influential they are in your life. First look close by. What made you do what you are doing right now? What made your day in the past? Then look further afield. What were the ingredients of the good times in your life? What was so rewarding then? What would be rewarding in the future? What do daydreams and phantasies tell you about your reinforcers when

you are lying idle? Grief, giving up and depression can also be understood in terms of reinforcement. When death takes away a loved one, all the reinforcers that were part of spending time together are gone, maybe irretrievably so. It's hard then to go on.

Reinforcers (read motivators) may not last forever. They may fade away once a goal has been reached. As Bernard Shaw put it so cogently: "It's easy to quit smoking. I have done it many times." It's easier to lose weight than to maintain weight loss. A new set of reinforcers is then required. Doing better with sports and socially might work, or a therapeutic dose of vanity.

Motivation is the Achilles heel of psychotherapy. An old joke describes it best: "How many psychiatrists does it take to change a light bulb? – Only one, but the bulb must really want changing." Motivation is also the Achilles heel of self-improvement. What motivates it? According to President G.H. Bush, it can be " the vision thing." It certainly sells lottery tickets. Imagine great riches coming your way, and spending a few bucks on buying a ticket comes easily. Improving quality of life consistently and persistently takes more effort. **Response cost** factors into the equation here. Not much will happen unless it's kept at a realistic level. Suppose you want to maintain a daily exercise quota. Suppose you also feel too worn and tired after work for a trip to the gym and pumping iron (read high response cost). A little **behavioral engineering** might overcome the impasse. Could you walk home part of the way or all the way? Exercising immediately after work eliminates procrastination. Walking home adds cheaper transport to your goal of daily exercise. Do you know someone you'd enjoy walking with? If so, you lowered your net response cost by adding pleasure (a reinforcer). Your response cost of not walking has also risen, assuming you don't want to let down your friend.

I would be badly amiss without including my "fourth office" in the streets of Toronto, the place where clients confronted fears and phobias head-on. **Exposure therapy** means what it says, exposure to feared situations. Preparations for the ordeal included coping techniques like calm breathing, relaxed posture and a reappraisal of faintness and palpitations as a normal part of exertion. I walked crowded streets, malls and rode the subway with agoraphobics from one end of the line to the other, spent hours in cars with road accident survivors and lunched on the top of high rises with height phobics. I borrowed cats from friends, snakes from pet shops and a supply of dead mice from the hospital lab to supplement my office equipment. *In vivo* exposure therapy was only a small part of my practice, but extremely worthwhile. It can quite literally "cure" a phobia. It also taught me more about panic anxiety than any description could.

One of my first clients ever was a **bird phobic**, too phobic even to know what a bird looked like close-up or how its feathers felt. I bought a mechanical bird that flapped its wings and made little squawking noises. Letting it loose in St. Mike's hospital hallways was marvelous fun, but ineffective. I tried loose feathers and a stuffed owl. This worked better. Once my client had managed to hold and stroke loose feathers and then the owl, we went for walks outdoors. She spotted birds from hundreds of yards away, even little ones. Would they swoop down and attack, replaying Hitchcock's movie "The Birds?" We discussed bird behavior and the fact that food and fear motivate them, not a creepy desire to attack in swarms. Success was defined as her ability to feed wild geese at Toronto Harbor. After conquering this, she visited local beaches and foreign shores. A postcard with a foreign stamp was proof of lasting success.

A **snake phobic** wouldn't go anyplace that had tall grass. Weekend cottages were off limits, as snakes might hide there. Tropical destinations were her dream, but completely out of reach. With some encouragement, she first handled a rubber snake, then a dead eel from Toronto's St. Lawrence Market. Then she was ready to face the real thing. I rented a mid-sized python from an obliging pet shop. Unbeknownst to her, I also hid a small ax under my couch before our first session with the snake, just in case. The snake was surprisingly strong when it wrapped itself around my arm. I decided against wrestling and guided it gently. I am better now. So is my client. She passed her ultimate test with a trip to a snake-ridden country in Southeast Asia. And I am on friendly terms with the milk snake in our basement. She even has a name.

A **spider phobic** wouldn't sleep in unfamiliar places and without her husband's presence. She searched her bedroom every night and with his help, to make absolutely sure no spider could possibly hide anywhere near her. It took some convincing before she agreed to look at the picture of a spider. Looking at a dead one came next, then touching it and eventually killing a live one, first with, and then without her husband's help. She had a trait in common with other phobics who dread small animals: She wanted to make absolutely certain that the critter could not catch her unawares. Learning to cope without assistance is crucially important in this regard. It's a recovering phobic's safeguard against relapse.

People with a variant of **obsessive-compulsive disorder** (OCD, aka contamination or germ phobia) outdo other phobics in wanting things predictable. Germs are too small for the naked eye. Someone with contamination phobia can never be sure if he has scrubbed thoroughly enough to eliminate the threat. He may scrub his hands raw, without ever feeling safe.

I applied three rules to the practice of exposure therapy:

*Never, ever spring a surprise on a phobic, like "voila, here's the mouse." Always let her approach her feared situation at her own pace, even if that takes hours. And never trap her.

*She must confront her fear without interruption once she has started exposure and keep at it for as long as it takes to extinguish her urge to leave. (Leaving early can make matters worse.) - Fight must win out over flight to guarantee success.

*Homework practice is needed after therapist-assisted exposure to make improvement stick, to produce sufficient *generalization* from one set of circumstances to all others that might apply. Without generalization, the client remains dependent of the therapist's presence. Repeated practice under varying conditions and in several places, first in the presence, then in the absence of the therapist is vital, to make improvement stick.

I used slides as a supplement to *in-vivo exposure*, slides of heights, planes and animals projected onto a wide screen to make them look as real as possible. The Canadian Broadcasting Corporation kindly provided soundtracks of thunderstorms and incoming artillery fire for other mock-ups. They were a pale pre-view of what's possible nowadays with the help of virtual reality. I sat comfortably in an easy chair a couple of years ago at the MASSMOCA museum, wearing a headset while flying high above a virtual New York City. Whenever I turned my head, my per-spective changed. I held on to my (real) seat to keep my balance, more so after the plane disintegrated in flight. That left only my seat between me and the skyscrapers of New York below. Debris and floating typewriters added in-flight entertainment. Virtual reality setups like this one cost money. They are cheap as a therapeutic aide, considering their potential benefits. Taking flight phobics on virtual plane rides, acrophobics on tall ladders and social phobics into virtual meetings will be more easily arranged with their help than in-vivo exposure. They will also save therapist time and increase access to treatment. - I wish I had a virtual environment of such quality for my practice.

Few challenges felt overwhelming. Given enough time, a solution could usually be found. Having to solve one problem after another for days on end could be stressful though. Fatigue would set in and with it the risk of making a mistake. When basic information about a new client's medications was missing and the client didn't have a clue, I could feel tension rise. It meant searching the pharmaceutical reference manual for a picture of the "little white pill" he might be taking, a time-waster that tightened a tight schedule even more. Here's a brief primer on how to do better:

Most **medications** have both a *generic* (e.g. Alprazolam) and a *trade name* (e.g. Xanax). Remember both, particularly when travelling, also the dosage. Here are more **must-knows**: All drugs have *side effects.* Recognizing them for what they are may save needless worries about a non-existing illness. Drugs also *interact with each other.* Some love each other and augment each other's effects. Others hate each other and diminish each other's effects. Some hate each other to the point of *contra-indication,* something your pharmacist will explain. Drugs also have a *half-life.* That's the time your system takes to eliminate 50% of them from your blood stream. Some half-lives are short, measured in hours. Others (like Prozac) last days, even weeks. Suppose your blood pressure medication has a half-life of twelve hours. Its blood level (and its therapeutic effect) may gyrate considerably if you take both pills together, just once a day. It will gyrate less if you take them separately, half a day apart. And there is *"bioavailability:"* A drug has to be absorbed by your gut and get from there into your blood stream, to be available. Some gut contents can interfere with drug absorption. If you washed it down with grapefruit juice or an antacid, it will be poor. And so will be the drug's effectiveness. - Ask your doctor and your pharmacist for details.

This much about therapy. How about the therapist? I faced a common dilemma. Should I spend more time on short-term therapy and prioritize patients who would get better fast? Or should I spend more time on open-ended care, emphasize the "caring" aspects of my appointments and see more chronic patients, with the unintended side effect of treating fewer patients that would benefit rapidly from therapy. Obviously, that's a matter of balance, but one that isn't arranged with ease, if you have a heart. A cartoon from Punch magazine may illustrate this. It portrays a wise man, skinny, in rags and with a long straggly beard. He's perched on a rocky promontory, cross-legged, straight upright and looking uncomfortable. Near him crouches his disciple, looking equally haggard. "Master," he implores, "how do you keep so calm?" "Well," speaks the master, "I scream a lot." Guarding my priorities and my schedule, participating in research and practicing several sub-specialties may have saved me from the master's fate. I never took a medical journal to the beach. And the Canadian Shield with its granite rocks warmed by the sun took care of stress and fatigue.

Consults at Anxiety disorders were usually assigned by roster. One day, a patient asked for me by name, even if that meant waiting a bit longer. I obliged, feeling flattered. He seemed satisfied after our therapeutic chat. But then, on his way out the door he turned back and asked: "Are you really Dr. Kuch?" Puzzled, I pointed to my nametag. He was unconvinced. "Well," he said, "you are ok. But I really wanted to see the Pakistani doctor." A Pakistani doctor with my name? I had to check. A second look at his chart reassured me that I had indeed seen him before. And then it dawned on me: His first visit had been in the summer. Now it was the middle of winter, and I no longer matched the nut-brown looks of "the Pakistani doctor."

Summer weekends in Ontario's North take me back to balmy Florida and breezy California, to smoky fires, board shorts, bare feet, morning coffee by the water and my second calling of just hanging loose. For years a second-hand Chevy Impala '64 convertible was part of the scene. I had bought it in Florida and loved to bits. It was black, had a white ragtop, red leather seats and a bench in the rear as wide as a family sofa. It had eaten many miles and "survived a good many wars," as a grease monkey put it after a patch-up. It also matched the longish hair and Zapata moustache I sported at the time. And so it happened that I rode it southbound on HIWY 400 after a long summer weekend. I was driving top down, wind in my hair and looking a little worse for wear when a police cruiser pulled up beside me. I slowed to the speed limit and kept studiously to my lane. The two cops in the cruiser eyeballed me for a while, then thumbed me over. Dutifully, I pulled onto the curb and stopped, feeling slightly guilty as I always do when I see a cop. One got out of the cruiser and ordered me out as well. He demanded car papers. I produced them. "Walk around the car," he commanded. I obliged. He studied my papers again, and for a long time, then pointed at my MD license plates (indicating a licensed Ontario physician). Looking me hard in the eye, he asked: "Are you a doctor." I assured him I was and produced my Medical Association card. He gave me a long thoughtful look, then turned to his partner in the cruiser. "I guess it must be true," he said. And with that they drove off.

19. THE RANT

We have lived through two years of pandemic misery by now, and everyone feels on edge. We are tired of masks, tests, social distancing and washing our hands for as long as it takes to sing the national anthem. Most of us have taken the jab. Most of us carry a vaccination pass. We have been good, but new variants keep popping up all the same. Social networks continue to dwindle. Dining out is still a nervous pleasure. Travel remains an obstacle course. And a bucolic scene like the one below from a Sicilian town looks like a thing of the past.

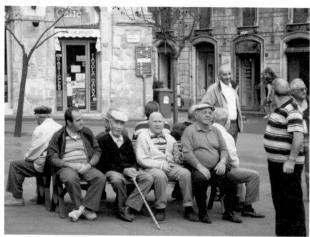

Sicilian market square

An antique German etching pictures life as an arc spanning the four seasons, spring, summer, fall and winter. Each step represents another decade. Tasks and challenges define each stage, as Eric Ericson tells us, from potty training to learning to walk and talk, onwards to finding friends, establishing a career and raising difficult children. At the age of fifty, we peak. And in old age, we repeat most developmental steps in reverse, all the way back to diapers and falling over. By the end, "God's grace is your only hope."

It's no surprise then that old guys get grumpy, considering what there is to look forward to.

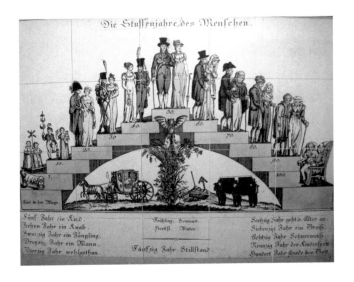

The Stages of Life; Haller Stadtmuseum

The pandemic augments these life challenges. New virus variants, overstretched health care services, global warming, mass migrations, inflation and economic uncertainty add to them, evoking feelings of anger, frustration, anxiety and doom. Epidemiologists report rising rates of anxiety, depression and substance use worldwide. A mental health crisis is grafting itself onto a virus pandemic.

Much of this is self-inflicted.

We have the vaccines, but close to one quarter of the general population remains stubbornly unvaccinated. Some pretend that the pandemic doesn't exist. Some worry, doubt, procrastinate and protest against a remedy that could save us from a lot of trouble. What can we do? Riding out the pandemic looks risqué when case numbers rise exponentially. Slowing it with lockdowns damages livelihoods and the economy. And vaccine mandates meet with vociferous protest. It's a three-way conflict, accentuated by fear and urgency. Should we hope for a mutation that makes COVID more like the common flu? Should we try mandates and lockdowns to safeguard hospital capacity and forestall even nastier variants, risking protest and confrontation in the process?

Some vaccine hesitants may be forgiven, the *needle phobics* who feel faint when they face an injection, the *illness phobics* who fear most things medical and the genuinely *paranoid* who can't help but see conspiracies everywhere. It's harder to understand the rest, the ones who resist obvious solutions. Why are they so reluctant?

Prevention is hard to sell at the best of times. Its costs, rules and inconveniences are up-front and in your face, the risks of doing nothing visible only to those who read the health statistics. The pandemic has us in its grip because there's no feedback loop, nothing to alert the incredulous to danger. You can't see the virus a N-95 mask just fended off like an efficient goalie. You can't see it multiply like the debt on your maxed-out credit card. You don't see the 5 ½ million people that died globally from COVID (WHO). Many doubters would run like scalded cats to the nearest clinic if they couldn't breathe the moment they encountered the virus. Instead, they "aren't sure," they "wait and see" and take their chances with their health as well as ours. And after vaccines have prevented the worst and the crisis has passed, they may well insist that it wasn't much of problem after all. A post-hoc comparison between vaccinated and unvaccinated COVID death rates would be convincing. Would they read it?

Scientific illiteracy may be a big part of this. How many in the general public recognize baseless scares and fake cures? How many understand COVID statistics in sufficient detail, as percentages of the underlying population? (remember the base-rate fallacy?) How many are familiar with drug and vaccine development and the safeguards that guarantee safety and efficacy? How many recognize a placebo when they see one on a drug store shelf? Patent medicines and dubious cures sell well. Health gurus hold sway over a multitude of followers. In some places, questioning false the utility of homeopathy comes close to offending religious sentiment.

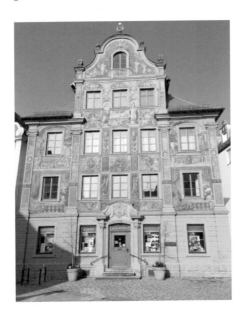

A German pharmacy and homeopathy

Scientific illiteracy is fertile ground for vague doubt and misinformation. Were COVID vaccines" released too soon?" That's a dead-end question. Scientific literacy means knowing how to ask actionable questions. "What should be done before release that hasn't been done" would be actionable, also "show me the data." Here are some data: Roughly 63% of all Americans have been fully vaccinated by the date of writing (January 22, 2022; usafacts.org), some 90% in the UK, 85% in China, 78% in Canada and 73% in Germany. Roughly 10 billion doses have been administered world-wide. Fatality rates have dropped massively amongst the vaccinated, and adverse effects are rare (ourworldindata.org). Overwhelmingly, the evidence supports full participation in approved vaccination programs.

I ran into a demonstration against vaccine mandates recently in Toronto. Out in front of a shivering crowd walked a young man with a bullhorn, shouting slogans about "freedom." Another one followed behind, shouting more of the same. Some two hundred marchers traipsed in between the two, placards declaring "my body is my right" and "no discrimination." I felt tempted to do a little shouting myself, ask if their "rights" carried any corresponding obligations, if they felt "free" to put others at risk and "free" to to hog hospital beds when COVID makes them ill. Concerns about civil liberties and excessive regulation have a rightful place in the vaccine debate. A prescription shouldn't cause more trouble than the illness it intends to prevent. Governments have done some ghastly things in the past, like eugenics and the Tuskegee experiments with syphilis in the American South. They have mis-informed, dis-informed, over-reacted, over-reached and made false promises. Officials have ignored their own health advisories and doubted them publicly. Doubt and asking for a mandate's rationale is good. Vague suspicion is not. Doubt and suspicion need to be as specific and as actionable as claims of vaccine benefits. They are useless otherwise and can't be followed up by independent oversight, by citizen sleuths or a free press. And those allegedly responsible can't be held accountable by parliament or the legal system. Vague suspicions and conspiracy theories only gum up the works.

No debates took place between the protesters I observed in Toronto and the surrounding crowd. They, just like the Ottawa truckers, looked like a self-isolating group, quarantined not from the virus but from differing opinion. Discussion ceases when the shouting starts and police are needed to keep demonstrators in check. Ideological isolation takes a hold then. And that produces another dynamic, **group think**. Enter Gustave LeBon's "Psychology of Crowds" (21): Individuals make better decisions on their own than they would as members of an isolated, close-knit group. Joining such a group requires conformity. Add the algorithm of social media that brings together likeminded with like-minded, and you have growth. Add the cherrypicking of news and an admiration for sloganeering, and you get mass protest with bullhorns and trucks.

How can we restore calm and dialogue? Debating restrictive measures with a reference to data could be one way. One-on-one debunking has also been suggested, this in regards to conspiracy theories that portray government as ill-willed (22): Could a policy error be a cock-up instead of a conspiracy? Wouldn't there be at least one whistleblower amongst the many who had to know about a fake epidemic dreamt up by civil servants? Wouldn't citizen-sleuths like *bellingcat* (23) ferret this out? Changing a true believer's convictions is hard. He hasn't requested your help. He isn't your client. And you are asking him to leave his spiritual home.

What else can penetrate a wall of incomprehension? Government is having a go at it by **imposing a cost on non-compliance**. It has done this for years with speeding, drunk driving and other kinds of malfeasance that endanger the public good. Remember Typhoid Mary, the asymptomatic cook and carrier of typhoid fever that infected her customers? She wouldn't cooperate with quarantine and had to be committed to an isolation center. By comparison, vaccine passports are minimally restrictive. They increase vaccination rates and save lives, as recent data from Europe indicate (The Economist). You can get a passport at the price of two harmless jabs. What alternative do the protesters have to offer?

20.BEFORE I GO

I retired from medical practice in stages and with regret. The Pain Clinic got the chop after my friend and mentor Ray Evans retired. Next came Anxiety Disorders and my home office. Forensics and a mood disorders clinic at the Royal Victoria Hospital in Barrie came last. Many good-byes happened on the way. My "failures" had stayed with me for years. They knew little about me personally, but there was a bond. I was walking away from patients who had depended on me for years. I called in old favors to refer them elsewhere; but it felt sad. One old-timer took a cutting from an office plant as a memento. Others were tearful. A few traveled almost a hundred miles north to the Royal Victoria Hospital to continue seeing me during my last two years of practice. And then I shut it all down and took my seat "in God's waiting room," as Ray used to call it. All of a sudden I had time on my hands, time for memories and time for thoughts about death and dying. And then I realized that this was another chance for a tilt at the windmills.

My father died from a heart attack when he was only 55 years old. His first infarct struck him in the middle of a November night. An ambulance took him to the hospital. I was at his bedside within hours and spent the next week there, hunched over textbooks for my medical boards. The window of his hospital room looked out over the river and the hills where we had spent so much time together. He described the pain he had felt in his chest during that fateful night, "sharp and severe like severing a finger." He was determined to recover and looked forward to the woods and the river. His condition stabilized and I returned to Heidelberg, to focus on my studies. I had been there for only a few days when a telegram arrived at the student residence. My dad had suffered a second infarct. A strange sense of detachment took over as I gathered up essential study materials, then left Heidelberg, speeding through evening gloom and rain. Ominously, an elevator waited for me at the ground floor of the hospital with its doors open. Dad was in the same room as before. Pillows supported his neck and head, keeping him half upright to ease his labored breathing. An IV was running. Oxygen-conducting tubes were in his nose. He was agitated, claustrophobic and fought off an oxygen tent. He had been giving last instructions to my step-mom until confusion overtook him. I held his hand, felt his racing pulse and looked into his terrified eyes. He struggled and shifted, seemingly unable to recognize me. Hours passed. His pulse grew fainter and ever more irregular, his breathing increasingly strained. His agony continued until close to midnight, when his doctor told us that all hope was lost. He rapidly pushed the contents of a syringe into a vein. My father's lips moved a few more times, mimicking breath. Then came the hiss of oxygen being disconnected, followed by silence. - I had witnessed an assisted death.

Another experience made me think about assisted death, this one decades later and very different. I was assessing an elderly lady in a large nursing home in regards to a compensation claim. The staff were exceptionally kind, the building spacious and clean. And it horrified me. The large entrance hall was well lit by a glass dome, but it lacked a view to the outside. Some twenty inmates sat there, slumped in wheelchairs that had been arranged in a semi-circle. An eerie silence reigned as all eyes followed me. Boredom was palpable. I was the event of the day. I found my client in bed in a room with curtains drawn. She was disoriented and terrified by my intrusion. A life-size doll was her only consolation, regardless of staff's efforts to reassure her. Her condition was chronic, but not life threatening. It condemned her to wait until death would release her. - I was visiting my own personal nightmare.

Both my dad and the above-mentioned lady didn't have a choice. In a sad way dad was lucky. His doctor took pity on him and saved him from slow asphyxiation by pulmonary edema, if only at the last minute. The old lady was just as helpless. She had no relief forthcoming. She'll be either bored silly or terrified and confused for as long as she's be alive. I have known several others who endured their last years in similar ways while wishing they were dead. And they were the lucky ones, the ones who were getting decent care. I hate to think of the others. Which gets me to Dying with Dignity (DwD), a Canadian charitable organization with sister organizations in many countries and more than a few battles for medical assistance in dying (MAID) under its belt. I hope that my doctor will save me from lengthy agony and from ending up helpless and bored silly in a nursing home. I am putting this request into my Advance Care Directive.

The Western world decriminalized suicide decades ago as part of a larger trend that has given people more rights over their body. Pain relief obtained priority over prolonging life years ago (WHO guidelines for palliative care). The administration of large doses of potent pain relievers is acceptable even when it hastens death. Switzerland, Belgium and the Netherlands went further and decriminalized MAID (medically assisted dying), followed by a growing number of US States, Canada and most recently Austria. Precautions are in place to ensure informed consent as an absolutely vital requirement before MAID, but the battle isn't over yet. In Canada it continues to rage over rules and precautions and over the attempts of the faithful to restrict access to MAID as much as possible. In several other countries MAID still attracts a criminal charge. To take the utilitarian view, why limit personal choice on a continent where "minding your own business" is a stock phrase and no harm results from it to the community?

Current Canadian legislation has overcome a good many hurdles, including the "Hobson's Choice" of someone with progressive dementia: Go to Switzerland for a needlessly early demise, or wait until loss of competence bars you from travel and from giving informed consent. A "reasonably foreseeable death" in the near future is no longer a requirement for MAID. At the time of writing, Canadian Law does not address another intricate matter, the intolerable suffering of competent persons who suffer exclusively from a mental illness that's beyond remediation. We strive to improve quality of life. We must strive to improve quality of death as well.

How does one outfox the prospects of life ending in one huge downer? That's not the way to end a book or a life. How does one maintain quality of life right up to the end? I plan to have fun the way I always had until the music stops, with as few concessions to age as possible, tilt at a few more windmills like home care and a more science-oriented discourse over public health measures. I want to champion openness, mutual support that reaches beyond borders and the mobility of talent. They should be available to others as they were to me, so they too can make their own way without hindrance.

Over to you.

ABBREVIATIONS

APA   American Psychiatric Association
CAMH   Center for Addiction and Mental Health
CPA   Canadian Psychiatric Association
DSM   Diagnostic Statistical Manual
ECFMG   Educational Council for Foreign Medical Graduates
EEG   Electroencephalography
KZ   *Konzentrationslager* (concentration camp)
LMCC   Licentiate of the medical Council of Canada
MAID   Medical Assistance In Dying
MAO   Monoamine Oxidase Inhibitor
OCD   Obsessive-compulsive Disorder
PTSD   Posttraumatic Stress Disorder
TB   Tuberculosis
UHN   University Health Network
VA   Veterans' Administration
WHO   World Health Organization

REFERENCES & RECOMMENDATIONS

1. Kenneth Colby (2014). Psychoanalysis and human behavior. Routledge

2. William Glassner (1965). Reality therapy. Harper & Row

3. Eric Fromm (2001). A Sane Society. Routledge

4. Karen Horney (1994). The neurotic personality of our time. WW Norton & Co

5. Eric Berne (2021). Games People Play; Amazon

6. Frederic S. Perls (1992). Gestalt therapy verbatim. Amazon

7. Arnold P. Goldstein (1973). Structured Learning Therapy: A Psychotherapy for The Poor. Academic Press, New York

8. Andrew Malleson (1973). The Medical Runaround. Hart Publishing Company

9. Claire Weekes (1969) Hope and Help for your Nerves. Berkley

10. Romeo Dallaire and Samantha Power (2004). Shake Hands with the Devil. Amazon

11. Anne Appelbaum (2003). Gulag: A History. Amazon

12. Daniel J. Levitin A Field Guide to Lies, Penguin Canada 2016

13. Derek Rowntree (1981). Statistics without tears: An Introduction to Non-Mathematicians. Ally & Bacon

14. June Callwood (1995). Trial without End. Alfred Knopf, Canada

15. M. Harris (1995) The Judas Kiss, Amazon

16. Isaac Meyer Marks (2005). Living with Fear. Paperback; McGraw-Hill

17. Mark Antony, Michele Graske and David Barlow (2006). Mastering your Fears and Phobias; Workbook; Oxford University Press

18. B.F Skinner (1965). Science and human behavior. Free Press

19. Steven Levitt and Stephen Dubner (2014). Think Like A Freak. Harper Collins

20. Tim Harford (2006). The Undercover Economist. Oxford University Press

21. Gustave Le Bon (2009). The Psychology of Crowds. Amazon

22. P. Harrison (2012). 50 Popular Beliefs that people think are true. Prometheus Books, Amherst

23. Eliot Higgins (2021). We are Bellingcat. Bloomsbury

Most of Klaus Kuch's refereed publications and citations can be found on www.researchgate.net and www.semanticscholar.com

ABOUT THE AUTHOR

Klaus Kuch

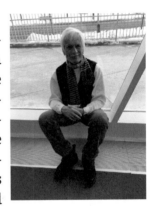

qualified as a general practitioner in Germany and Canada, in the US and Canada also as a psychiatrist. He is a member of the American Psychiatric Association (inactive) and the Canadian Psychiatric Association (life). His special interests include behavioral and cognitive therapies for phobias, PTSD and pain, also forensics. His publications on these subjects have gained international recognition.

He practiced at St. Michael's Hospital, Toronto General Hospital and the Center of Addiction and Mental Health at the University Health Network in Toronto, also at the Royal Victoria Hospital in Barrie, Ontario. He was a part-time associate professor at the University of Toronto with a cross-appointment in Anesthesia. He consulted on behalf of the Ontario Workplace Safety and Insurance Board (WSIB), its Appeals Tribunal, the Ontario College of Physicians and Surgeons, the Consulate General of Germany, Ontario's Crown Law Office and numerous law firms in civil and criminal litigation cases.

He is retired, married, lives on a farm, is intermittently interested in sports and keeping chickens but refuses to have anything to do with serious farm work.

He may be reached at

https://www.linkedin.com/
oldbones345@bell.net

Manufactured by Amazon.ca
Bolton, ON